BEAT UNWANTED WEIGHT GAIN

BEAT UNWANTED WEIGHT GAIN

(7 Ways to Lose Pounds and Never Regain Them)

John M. Poothullil, MD, FRCP

Over and Above Creative

IMPORTANT NOTICE

This book is not intended to replace the care of a physician. It also presents a new explanation on the cause and reversal of high blood sugar and Type 2 diabetes. The recommendations provided can help a reader with high blood sugar or Type 2 diabetes. If you follow them, we suggest you work with your physician as you lose weight and lower your blood sugar.

Editorial Direction and Editing: Rick Benzel Creative Services
Additional Editing: Robin Quinn
Copyediting: Julie Simpson, OnWords & UpWords!
Cover and Book Design: Susan Shankin / Precocity Press

Published by Over and Above Creative, Los Angeles, CA

ISBN: 978-0-9971077-2-2 (Trade paper)
ISBN: 978-0-9971077-3-9 (eBook)

Printed in China

CONTENTS

INTRODUCTION

Thank you for picking up this book. I'd like to start by asking you some questions.

Have you been struggling to lose weight, or to stop yourself from gaining more? Is being heavier than you would like making you feel uncomfortable, unattractive, or unhealthy? Do you wish you could finally shed some pounds and wear clothes that you used to wear? Do you worry about never being able to lose weight?

If you've answered "yes" to any of these, I hope you'll read this entire book and follow the advice I will provide. I truly want to help anyone who's seeking ways to beat unwanted weight gain.

Let me say immediately that this is not a "fat-shaming" book. I will not tell you how much weight you should lose or what you should look like. People come in all sizes and shapes because our human evolution goes back hundreds of thousands of years. We each have a family ancestry and genetic inheritance that has determined whether we are tall or short, heavyset or thin, big- or small-boned.

But your genes and family history don't dictate everything about your weight. If you've decided you're gaining too much or weigh more than you want to, there is something in your consciousness telling you it's time to change. That's a good sign. It means you're aware of how your weight impacts your health and your life. It also means you're open to listening to weight loss advice without feeling insulted or hurt. It especially means you have a good chance of successfully conquering the challenges ahead.

I cannot overstate the benefits of preventing unwanted weight gain. It has been known for some time that excessive weight gain is associated with about 200 illnesses. These include diabetes, cancer, heart failure, and premature death. It is also known that if unwanted weight gain is prevented or reversed, many of these conditions improve or disappear.

Carrying too much weight has many harmful health consequences. Excessive weight gain is associated with about 200 illnesses.

The Forces Against Your Desire to Lose Weight

I congratulate you on starting a journey with this book to beat your unwanted weight gain. But let me help you be totally realistic about what's in front of you, as there are a lot of potential roadblocks that might make you turn back from your commitment. Consider these:

1. As you start to make the recommended changes, you might wonder what the big deal is about being overweight or obese. Does it really matter to anyone? Why should you care about your weight?

These are important issues to think about correctly. Many people abandon the struggle with weight by concluding it doesn't matter. Let me tell you something: *It does matter.* Carrying too much weight has many harmful health consequences. Plus, being heavier than what's appropriate for your body can lower your energy, your productivity, and your general level of fitness.

For many people, feeling overweight affects their mental health, their sense of self-esteem, and their confidence around other "normal weight" people. Being overweight can lead to obesity (meaning body fat to weight ratio is over 30%), the consequences of which can be severe. Obesity is associated with many illnesses. For one, obese people are at a greater risk of developing Type 2 diabetes, which can lead to loss of vision, kidney problems, neuropathy, and even limb amputation. In short, being overweight should matter to you, and I hope you don't abandon a commitment to losing weight because you think it doesn't matter.

2. In your journey to lose weight, you'll likely be surrounded by family, friends, and strangers who are unlike you, either because they are genetically predisposed to remaining at a healthy weight without, apparently, needing to work at it, or because they're overweight but not interested in losing pounds. In fact, a study published in the medical journal *The Lancet* in November 2024 indicates that weight gain in the U.S. has been increasing for three decades.[1] Nationwide, nearly

1. https://www.nytimes.com/2024/11/14/well/obesity-epidemic-america.html

75% of adults over 25 are overweight (BMI greater than 25) or obese (BMI over 30). But don't let this be a roadblock; the fact that the majority of Americans are overweight has nothing to do with your personal desire to take control of *your own* weight.

You may even encounter people who try to get you to give up your commitment to losing weight, perhaps because they themselves are overweight or may consider you to be too slim compared to them. Some family and friends truly enjoy having meals with you and would like you to eat as much as they do. Or they want to know you enjoy their cooking and so they encourage you to eat second and third helpings. When this happens, what I suggest you do is to thank them and tell them you have no doubt that their cooking is delicious, and you have enjoyed it before. If you feel you must, take a small bite to oblige the host. But you'll need to tell these folks that you are beginning to feel good about losing some pounds and intend to follow through on your plan to get back in control of your weight. You can mention that you read this book and are feeling inspired and motivated to live a healthier lifestyle.

You may encounter people who try to get you to give up your commitment to losing weight . . . You'll need to learn to tell them you intend to follow through on your plan.

In today's social media environment, your commitment to losing weight may also be weakened whenever you spend time with friends who love meeting up at restaurants and bars, posting photos of everyone having a great time. Hanging out with them might tempt you to eat and drink as much as they do, and so you find it hard to say no. But here again, you need to honor your plan to lose weight and take better care of yourself. Remember, you are in charge of how much you eat, so enjoy being with your friends but keep your promise to yourself.

3. Although you desire to lose weight, you'll face a culture that is antithetical to people eating a healthy diet. For instance, everywhere you go there will be fast-food restaurants. You'll be tempted to buy their meals out of convenience when you're in a rush. They've learned how to make their food look good, appearing to also taste good, while most are often extremely high in calories, carbohydrates, and salt. Some restaurants offer all-you-can-eat buffets, and others serve huge portions that will entice you to double or triple the amount of food you need to eat at a single sitting.

   Meanwhile, grocery stores will present you with aisle after aisle of attractively packaged foods that call out to you to purchase them. You can easily get hooked on many of these products (if you're not already); in reality, they contain ingredients that contribute to your weight gain. I will show you how to read food labels so you can make better choices about what to buy at the supermarket.

   As you work on your weight, you'll learn how to resist eating at too many restaurants or, when you do, ordering unhealthy meals that put on pounds. You'll also learn how to make better choices at grocery stores.

4. Finally, you'll encounter scores of articles on the internet and in your social media feeds that will try to convince you that you can lose weight using some type of diet or program. As you'll learn in this book, I don't believe in or endorse any of these—and for good reason. Research has shown that nearly everyone who follows a third-party corporate diet program or buys pre-measured meals, despite initially losing some weight, in the end almost always regains it. When it comes to programs such as fasting and alternate-day eating, I suggest that these can cause your body to miss out on obtaining the nutrients your cells need for proper functioning. This is why many people become tired or lose productivity when they follow such programs.

> **Grocery stores will present you with aisle after aisle of attractively packaged foods . . . in reality, they contain ingredients that contribute to your weight gain.**

Learning to eat right to maintain a healthy weight must come from inside you in all regards. Developing the self-knowledge and the willpower to lose weight is ultimately your responsibility. This book will teach you how to develop those skills.

Using Drugs to Lose Weight Is Not the Answer

Before you read on, I need to address the newest trend in weight loss: the use of prescription drugs. Many of these medications were created for other medical purposes but were found to help people lose weight. Despite the highly touted success that some celebrities have had shedding pounds while taking such drugs, I don't recommend medications as a healthy long-term solution. As a physician, I know that relying on drugs to treat certain conditions does not ultimately solve the problem. In the case of weight gain, using pharmaceuticals does not teach you how to eat the right amount of food for your body, nor which foods are best to avoid weight gain.

Most importantly, relying on a medication to maintain weight control for the rest of your life has its risks. Medical science doesn't yet know the long-term effects of many of these drugs. Pharmaceutical companies sometimes have to withdraw a drug that turned out to be life threatening. One such instance occurred in the late 1990s. Two decades earlier, the drug fenfluramine was being used as a weight loss drug, but it was not very effective. In the early 1990s, doctors began combining it with phentermine. The combination was popularly known as fen-phen. However, in 1997, fenfluramine was cited as causing pulmonary hypertension and heart valve problems and had to be withdrawn from the market. This is just one example of how a drug believed to be useful turned out to be dangerous for patients years later.

Medications are not a healthy long-term solution. Using drugs does not teach you how to eat the right amount of food for your body, nor which foods are best to avoid weight gain.

In short, I don't recommend relying on drugs as your long-term solution to the problem of unwanted weight. The information in this book will show you a safer, more effective permanent path to a slimmer and healthier you.

HOW WEIGHT LOSS DRUGS WORK

Some weight loss drugs in use today are largely variants of medications used to treat convulsions, addiction, or depression that were also found to lower appetite. Others are modifications of drugs used to lower blood sugar in Type 2 diabetes. This latter type of drug works as follows. Normally, the intestine releases a hormone in response to glucose molecules in food. This hormone stimulates the pancreas to release insulin, but it also suppresses the sensation of hunger for a short time. With these new drugs, researchers have found a way to prolong the action of this intestinal hormone to achieve continued insulin release and thus a longer suppression of hunger. You don't feel like eating as much. This may seem like a good way to eat less, but it is not.

The danger is that some weight loss drugs can be addictive and cause severely high blood pressure if taken for a long period of time. The Type 2 diabetes drugs modified for weight loss have been found to cause nausea, vomiting, diarrhea, and

The Seven Ways to Lose Pounds and Never Regain Them

Are you ready to begin your exciting journey to lose some pounds? Some of my advice is common sense, but I also offer you many new insights based on verifiable scientific fact. But don't worry; even if you haven't studied biology in decades—or ever—I believe you'll be able to understand the explanations.

Here is an overview of the seven ways to permanently reverse unwanted weight gain. Each is discussed in one of the next seven chapters.

constipation in a significant number of people. Clearly, people with an upset stomach will eat less food and so lose weight. The prolonged suppression of hunger by weight loss drugs may also interfere with the intake of needed nutrients in a timely fashion, leading to food cravings. Worse, the continued release of insulin could lead to cancer cell growth. Finally, the potential complications associated with long-term use of these drugs have not yet been fully identified.

In most cases of drug-induced weight loss, the rate at which one loses weight tapers off significantly after about one year. Whether from discouragement or other reasons, when people stop taking the drug they start regaining the weight.

Many non-prescription food supplements are also being marketed as natural weight loss products, but they lack long-term controlled studies for verification. There is also no standardization of strength or quality control measures. Some are known to produce insomnia, irritability, and headache.

In short, you are taking a chance when you resort to medications or food supplements as your method to lose weight.

1. Reconnect with Your Authentic Weight

I won't tell you how many pounds to lose. That is up to you to determine. In Chapter 1, I provide you with some interesting guidance regarding how you can decide how much you ideally want to weigh. It's called reconnecting with your "authentic weight."

2. Identify Why You Overeat

In this chapter I help you identify the five reasons you might be overeating when you're not truly hungry. Once you understand your patterns, you'll become better at not overeating.

3. Pay Attention to the Signals of Hunger and When to Stop Eating

People who gain weight are often out of touch with their body's natural signals of hunger and satiation (satisfaction). So in Chapter 3, I remind you how to notice the real signals of hunger and explain how your body tells you when you have eaten enough.

4. Break Your Old Eating and Food-Shopping Habits

You've been eating your meals a certain way for decades, right? So how do you begin making changes to establish healthier habits? In this chapter, I explain how you can change the neural patterns in your brain that keep you locked into your old habits. We'll look at changing how you shop for food, how you store it in your home, and even how to make your portion sizes more appropriate to avoid weight gain.

5. Reduce Your Consumption of Grain-Based Carbs

What most people don't know is that grains and grain-flour products are the real culprits in weight gain. It's not the sugar you put in your coffee that puts on those pounds, neither is it the fat in meat or dairy. It's the wheat, barley, oats, corn, and rice—and the flours made from those grains—that fill your fat cells. Chapter 5 explains why you must reduce your consumption of carbohydrates—e.g., breads, rolls, pastries, pizza, pasta, rice, corn, tortillas, muffins, doughnuts, cakes, etc.—to lose weight.

6. Eat for Good Health, and to Feel Great

If you're going to change your eating habits, a guiding principle is to eat to be healthy. I explain in this chapter several elements of this eating lifestyle, including eating a diverse diet, learning how to read food labels, not relying on third-party corporate diets, avoiding no-calorie sweeteners, watching your alcohol consumption, feeding your good gut bacteria to build your immune system, and, finally, what I call "mindful eating."

What most people don't know is that grains and grain-flour products are the real culprits in weight gain.

7. Exercise to Stay Healthy, Not to Lose Weight

Many people believe that exercising will help them lose weight. However, this is a misconception. Most exercise doesn't burn off enough calories compared to what you consume in a day. So although it's possible that exercising may result in weight loss, it's not probable. And the older you get, it's even less likely. However, there are many good reasons you should exercise. Chapter 7 explains how exercise improves your overall health, which ultimately can lead to greater self-confidence about your body.

I hope you enjoy reading these chapters and that you will put my advice to use in your life.

(1)

RECONNECT WITH YOUR AUTHENTIC WEIGHT

The first step to beat unwanted weight gain is to figure out how much you should weigh. To start, you need a baseline weight to use when determining whether you are gaining weight or losing it. If you don't know this, here's what happens. Each year, you gain a pound or two (or more), and eventually you begin to think that this is now your weight. You lose sight year after year of what your real weight should be.

To combat that scenario, here's some encouraging news. Every person has access to a truly wise method for figuring out if they're too heavy and carrying too much body fat. It's what I call "rediscovering your authentic weight."

When I talk to people about this concept, almost everyone knows exactly what I mean. It's intuitive and immediate—and I assume many of you understood it as soon as you read it. This is similar to intuitively knowing what someone means when they talk about "justice," "equality," or "morality"—without their having to define it.

Perhaps you have never considered your authentic weight. Once you begin reflecting on it, you will likely get a good sense of what it should be. If you're being honest with yourself, you'll probably be able to know it without much hesitation. Reflect on it now. What would you say is your authentic weight?

Reconnecting with your authentic weight is the first step in getting back in control. When you are in tune with your authentic weight, you will immediately sense if you are gaining a few extra pounds. You'll know this because, admit it, you start to feel uncomfortable. Your stomach starts to feel bloated and distended; you may feel some muscle pains in your back. Or you may feel slower and more tired. Exceeding your sense of your authentic weight will be what prompts you to become aware that you need to lose some pounds. It will make you say to yourself, *Gee, I think I'm gaining weight.*"

Unfortunately, most people tend to rationalize their weight gain once they go beyond their authentic weight by a few pounds. They attribute it to stress, aging, busy days at work, family obligations, lack of time to exercise, or simply the fact that other people around them are also gaining weight. Such rationalization becomes increasingly convincing over time because your brain tends to believe ideas it repeats. Do you do this?

As you work with this book, reconnecting with your authentic weight will be the key to knowing how much weight you should strive for and maintain. We'll explore more about the concept later in this chapter and throughout the book.

Can't I Just Use Standardized Weight Tables?

You may wonder why you cannot just use the standard weight tables as a guide to determine your authentic weight. Let me explain why.

Most people tend to rationalize their weight gain. They attribute it to stress, aging, busy days at work, family obligations, or lack of time to exercise. Such rationalization becomes increasingly convincing over time because your brain tends to believe ideas it repeats. Do you do this?

There's something most people don't know about the most common weight guidelines used by U.S. doctors. Most of these tables are based on data originally obtained way back in 1943 from the Metropolitan Life Insurance Company (MetLife). MetLife was trying to calculate the insurance risk of people dying.

Policyholders were asked to self-report their height and weight when they purchased life insurance. MetLife then used that data to prepare a chart of "ideal" weights based on the lowest mortality rates among their customers. People who lived the longest were deemed to have been at an ideal weight at the age they were when they filled out the survey.

This means that the reported body weights were not verified by actual on-the-spot measurements to establish a definitive link between weight and mortality. As a result, these weight tables are effectively useless. Haven't you ever fibbed on a form?

In 1985, a new height and weight chart was prepared by the Gerontology Research Center, National Institute of Aging, Baltimore, Maryland. It attempted to calculate a healthy weight range for adults of all ages. Sounds promising, right?

Unfortunately, there are two main problems with this newer chart. First, the range of weights for each height is too broad. Second, it does not significantly help in predicting whether someone might develop a weight-related health problem. For example, there's no clear "cut-off" point in any weight range that determines what extra amount of weight triggers high blood sugar.

Let's say you are 35 years old, stand at 5 feet, 5 inches tall, and weigh 147 pounds. The 1985 height/weight chart says you are normal, as you fit inside the bracket between 115 and 149 pounds. But let's say that after developing prediabetes, you succeed at losing 12 pounds to weigh just 135 pounds, and your blood sugar returns to normal. How could you have known that your non-diabetic weight should have been at the lower end of the range rather than the higher?

What About Using Body Mass Index (BMI) to Know My Ideal Weight?

Some people use the ratio of body fat to weight as a guideline to determine how much they should weigh. One method to measure body fat is underwater weighing. The differences in density of fat, muscle, and bone allow an accurate determination of body fat. The problem? This method doesn't specify the amount of fat in each location of your body so it doesn't give a good clue as to where you might lose fat.

Another measure is the Body Mass Index (BMI), which is cheaper and faster. This measurement may be

HOW OFTEN SHOULD I WEIGH MYSELF?

I recommend people over age 35 check their body weight once a day at the same time. A good time is in the morning, for example, under the same conditions, such as after your first visit to the bathroom. This habit can help you become aware of weight changes before they're an issue. It will also help you identify what activities during the previous 24 hours contributed to any weight gain. Your goal is to maintain your body weight at your authentic weight, or less than 10 pounds above it. Making a note of your weight each day on a bathroom calendar or in a fitness app can assist in tracking how you're doing.

provided during visits to your primary care doctor. BMI is a little better than underwater weighing. It's based on a mathematically derived formula that considers the effect of your height on your body weight. More height generally means more bone and muscle, which weigh more than fat.

Statistics show that people who have a greater percentage of bone and muscle tend to have a lower BMI than those with a higher percentage of body fat. To find your BMI, you can go to the website for the National Heart, Lung, and Blood Institute and search "BMI." The search will take you to a BMI calculator where you can measure your own Body Mass Index. You'll also see where you fall on their scale from underweight to obese. How did you do?

Please note, however, the BMI test can be misleading. Its formula cannot distinguish fat mass from muscle mass. Muscle weighs more than fat because it is denser. If you are very muscular at any height, it adds to your weight, skewing your BMI. A test might indicate that you are overweight or obese, when, in fact, you are not.

Older readers should be aware of another problem with using BMI as a measure of what your weight should be. If you're an older person who has lost muscle, the BMI test may underestimate your body fat. Its formula assumes a certain amount of muscle for each height. So if you have lost muscle due to aging or lack of exercise, more of your weight will be stored as fat. This means your BMI might indicate that you are in the normal range when, in fact, you have too much fat and are likely overweight.

The BMI test can be misleading. Its formula cannot distinguish fat mass from muscle mass.

Formerly, a BMI between 25 and 30 meant you were overweight, while a BMI over 30 meant you were obese. Given the flaws of BMI, however, in June 2023 the American Medical Association suggested that BMI is not a good measure to define being overweight or obese. It does not help directly assess the effects of body fat mass on medical conditions such as hypertension and cardiovascular diseases for an individual. BMI also does not take into account the impact of any medical conditions, lifestyle issues, gender, ethnicity, familial conditions, and aging on one's health.

THE HEALTH CONSEQUENCES OF OBESITY

Being significantly overweight has potential consequences for your health. In particular, being obese can lead to many complications. So if you cannot use BMI to determine if you are overweight or obese, what information can help as you try to assess your authentic weight?

Here is my suggestion for how to understand obesity. While height is a function of bone length, one's total body weight is made up of many components, including fat, water, muscles, bones, and organs. Of all these components, the health complications associated with obesity are primarily related to the amount and distribution of fat (i.e., where it is located in your body). Given this, I propose that we can distinguish between ***cosmetic*** obesity and ***medical*** obesity.

- ***Cosmetic obesity*** occurs when the excess fat you maintain in your body is stored in your fat cells, not in your blood. This storage of fat does not usually cause medical complications. People with cosmetic obesity do not necessarily have to lose weight if they choose not to. However, cosmetic obesity can lead to emotional and self-esteem problems as you might be concerned about how other people look at you and interact with you. Also consider that, in some people, it can eventually create joint problems, such as with the ankles or knees.

- ***Medical obesity*** is more severe and occurs when some of the excess fat you maintain in your body stays in your blood either as triglycerides or as cholesterol, based on your genetic inheritance. The primary reason for this form of storage is that the fat cells in various locations in your body are nearly filled to capacity, so the excess fat remains in the blood. This can lead to medical conditions such as Type 2 diabetes and artery blockage that can cause stroke and heart disease. Not every person who has cosmetic obesity becomes someone with medical obesity, unless they entirely fill up their already elevated fat storage capacity. A person with medical obesity should strive to lose weight to avoid severe health complications.

You may have seen recent articles that say that obesity is a genetic condition, suggesting that some people cannot be held responsible for their weight or that they cannot lose weight even if they choose to. In my view, these articles describe ***cosmetic*** obesity, so let's understand this in more detail.

Why might someone be born and quickly become obese in childhood or early adulthood and remain obese throughout their lifetime? How could they be genetically predetermined to store a lot of fat? I believe that there are three potential explanations.

The first explanation is that fat is an excellent insulator for people who live in cold climates; they may store more fat to protect themselves. Some people may have had ancestors who lived in cold climates, and a genetic mechanism has therefore been transmitted from generation to generation continuing this form of fat storage, even when one generation moved to a warmer climate.

A second possible explanation for cosmetic obesity is that when people live in a region where the main source of food energy is poor in micronutrients, the body must consume more food, forcing it to store the extra energy as fat. This cause can also have become genetically inherited. As with ancestors who lived in cold climates, such a person's genetic heritage provided more fat storage capacity to keep fat away from the blood.

The third possibility for cosmetic obesity does not have to do with your distant ancestors, but with your mother. She may have consumed excess nutrition when you were developing inside her womb. As a result, you may have an excess of fat stem cells that have become fat storage as you grew into an adult.

This is not to suggest that if you are cosmetically obese, you should not consider losing weight. Keep in mind that even in cases of cosmetic obesity, you can eventually suffer health consequences by filling your fat storage capacity, leading to excess fat being kept in your blood. If you are cosmetically obese and want to lose weight, you can do so by following the guidelines in this book.

Are You Ready to Be Honest About Your Weight?

To avoid the many ill health effects related to being overweight, your goal must be to take back control of your body and rediscover your authentic weight. Obviously, you can look in the mirror and see whether you are carrying layers of fat in your abdomen, hips, or buttocks. If so, you need to be honest with yourself and admit that you would be healthier if you lost weight.

Your authentic weight is approximately the body weight you had when you were in your mid-twenties. However, be aware that aspects of your weight can change as you exercise and age, and your authentic weight will adjust.

So, here's the question. Are you unable to figure out what your authentic weight is?

If so, use this rule of thumb. Your authentic weight is approximately the body weight you had when you were in your mid-twenties, provided that you were not overweight, and your blood sugar and triglyceride levels were within normal range at that time. That is the age at which you probably reached your full height, and your bones reached their maximum density.

However, be aware that aspects of your weight can change as you exercise and age, and your authentic weight will adjust. For instance, have you been working out more? You may be adding muscle (which is denser than fat and can add weight). Interestingly, though you might be gaining muscle weight, your brain will know you are still in your authentic range. It takes into account your extra muscle mass.

Here's another helpful clue regarding staying in control of your authentic weight. If your health insurance covers an annual physical checkup that includes a battery of blood tests, the physician should check to see if your levels of triglycerides, blood glucose, and cholesterol are within the normal range in a fasting state. If you see your triglycerides, cholesterol, and/or blood sugar starting to rise, it means that you are moving outside of your authentic weight. It's time to pay more attention to what you're eating and how much of it. You could soon be on a slippery slope to obesity,

CAN I HAVE A SURGICAL PROCEDURE TO LOSE WEIGHT?

If you are thinking about getting bariatric (obesity) surgery to shed an extreme amount of weight, beware. The main types of bariatric surgery each have their pros and cons. Here's a quick review.

Some procedures reduce the ability of the intestines to absorb nutrients. Though this may help a person lose weight, it can result in deficiencies of iron, vitamin B12, fat-soluble vitamins, thiamine, and folate. Inappropriate insulin secretion is another complication of this type of surgery. Yet another is deep vein thrombosis with a potential for pulmonary embolism. In addition, rapid weight loss after obesity surgery can contribute to the development of gallstones.

Other procedures restrict your food intake by making the stomach smaller. The gastric bypass, for example, reduces the size of the stomach by well over 90%; that is, to about 15 milliliters (ml) in size compared to a normal stomach that can stretch, sometimes to over 1000 ml. What you may not realize is that this procedure helps you lose weight simply because you cannot eat as much as before. So before agreeing

Type 2 diabetes, and/or cardiovascular disease if you let your weight, blood sugar, and cholesterol rise too high. If your insurance does not cover such blood testing, you might find low-cost labs where you can obtain the tests.

You Can Do This!

You now have your first solution—knowing your authentic weight. Feel good about that. You have a targeted goal.

As you work with this book, you'll be establishing new behaviors to support achieving and maintaining your

to this type of surgery, I suggest you find out how much food someone who had this type of surgery can consume. Then, as an experiment, try eating a similar amount of food for a few weeks. See if you can achieve similar weight loss and weight maintenance without having to suffer the surgery and its consequences.

In short, the intended result of all the various bariatric surgeries is to reduce the amount of nutrients absorbed following a meal so that the quantity to be stored as fat is lessened, leading to reduced body weight. In practice, this result is attained by a combination of reducing the capacity of the stomach to accommodate incoming foods during a meal or by reducing the amount of nutrients that can be absorbed after meal.

However, here is a warning: After bariatric surgery, people may tend to feel good about themselves for the weight loss, but many of them experience psychological complications, including but not limited to grieving the loss of enjoying food, mourning the loss of the identity they had come to know as themselves, regrets about having had surgery, relationship changes, and fear of regaining weight.

authentic weight. This requires your commitment and determination. The positive news is that before long new eating behaviors will be firmly established. Then the plans in this book will become relatively easy for you to follow.

Whatever your current age, the recommendations in this book will help you age more healthfully. When you achieve your authentic weight, you will find yourself having more energy, feeling better about yourself, and finally enjoying one of the most meaningful activities of life—eating. Each meal will become a sensory experience that delights you and reinforces your ability to eat for nourishment and avoid excess food intake.

After bariatric surgery, people may tend to feel good about themselves for the weight loss, but many of them experience psychological complications.

Key Points

- Do you want to feel motivated to eat properly and avoid the foods that cause weight gain? The key to this is to become aware of your "authentic weight."
- Know that standardized weight tables, body-fat-to-weight ratios, and Body Mass Index (BMI) are all unreliable sources for your goal weight.
- Still need help grasping the concept of authentic weight? Try this guideline: Your authentic weight is approximately the body weight you had when you were in your mid-20s, provided you were not overweight and your blood sugar and triglyceride levels were within normal range at that time.

(2)

IDENTIFY WHY YOU OVEREAT

It's mid-morning and you're hard at work. The phone rings and you end up talking to a difficult client for 30 minutes. After you hang up, you're tense and you feel like you need something to eat, even though you had a big breakfast—two eggs, home fries, ham, and toast. Since you have to head out to do an errand anyway, you stop at a coffeehouse and get a large latte and a couple of big chocolate chip cookies. You deserve a treat after that tough conversation, right? Then you're back to the office for another hour of work, and it's lunchtime with a friend at a nearby pizza place.

Mid-afternoon, though, you can't stop thinking about that divine chocolate cake that the bakery down the street sells, so you head out and grab a slice. After another few hours of work, you join colleagues for a drink. The bar offers bowls of pretzels and nuts, plus free hors d'oeuvres, so you pile yourself a plateful.

Later that evening, it's dinner with the family. The chicken parmesan is so tasty you can't stop at one helping. *Why not?* you think, as you go for seconds. You are so full after dinner you decline dessert, deciding you really don't need to eat more today.

However, inexplicably, you get a craving for a peanut butter and jelly sandwich before bed, and you just can't help yourself from making one and eating it as you watch the late-night news before going to sleep.

Does this scenario remind you of your own eating habits? Are you indulging in food pretty much all day long, without ever thinking about whether you're actually hungry?

The fact is, people usually gain weight because they eat too often and too much. The body cannot use all the calories they consume, which causes the body to store the excess as fat.

This leads us to the second step for beating weight gain: identifying why you are overeating. I propose that there are five behavioral reasons people eat too much:

1. They eat for the pure enjoyment of food, even when they're not hungry.
2. They eat to relieve stress and anxiety.
3. They do eat only when they are hungry, but they overeat on a regular basis.
4. They eat while distracted.
5. They eat in response to clever food marketing.

If you tend to overeat, you probably do so for two or more of the above reasons. Do you resonate with any of these? Before you continue reading, jot down which reasons you suspect apply to you.

Are you indulging in food pretty much all day long, without ever thinking about whether you're actually hungry?

Whatever your reasons, you're overriding your brain's true hunger and satiation signals—natural signals from your body, which I'll discuss in the next chapter.

But now, let's examine these five reasons so you can better understand them.

Reason 1: Overeating for the Pure Enjoyment of Food

As an infant, toddler, and young child, you probably did not eat when you weren't hungry. Most young children tend to be completely in touch with their hunger and satiation signals. They may love the taste of certain foods, but they only eat when hunger drives them to do so and then only to the point of satisfaction.

I believe that non-hunger eating begins as a temporary and occasional accident, often in association with social events. It usually starts around your adolescent years and continues into adulthood. Social overeating is done without recognizing its long-range significance. For most people, it starts with certain events or situations—such as family picnics and holiday meals, or lunches and dinners out with friends. The pattern is reinforced as you begin eating different foods and experience new tastes, such as during an exciting meal at a flavorful ethnic restaurant.

I believe that non-hunger eating begins as a temporary and occasional accident, often in association with social events. It usually starts around your adolescent years and continues into adulthood.

The more such events occur, the more repetition reinforces the connection in the brain between eating and the enjoyment of great-tasting food. Whether you're hungry or not, if food is available and appealing to your taste buds, you learn to feel it's acceptable to eat a lot of it. You may sense that it's not appropriate to eat so much, but little by little you convince yourself that eating without being hungry can't be all that bad, especially if you're with family or friends. The pleasure of eating delicious food eventually overcomes your inclination to wait for the true sensation of hunger.

Over the years, your mind develops ways to rationalize the unwanted consequences of your budding overeating behavior. By the time you're in your mid- to late twenties, you may start to gain some weight. But you justify it by telling yourself, *It's just a few extra pounds and I can take it off easily.* You know that you're eating too much, but dismiss it by thinking, *I can stop doing this any time I want, but for now, I'm enjoying the food.* This pattern of eating is often strengthened by friends and family around you who are overeating too, thus encouraging, if not normalizing, the behavior.

A repetitive act is reinforced when it is accompanied by strong feelings. In this case, it is the pleasure associated with food or with a pleasurable event. You begin to establish a behavior of eating when stimulated by the sight, smell, or even just the thought of food, or a particular occasion or venue, rather than by your body's hunger signals. You love the feeling of enjoyment that delicious food gives you.

Once you reach this stage, your awareness of—or even the presence of—adverse long-term consequences may not be enough to correct your inability to stop overeating. The outcomes might include weight gain, high blood sugar, high blood cholesterol, or high blood pressure. But your behavior continues, even when the consequences are damaging.

This pattern of behavior regarding food is not unlike other "addictive" behaviors people can develop out of an inability to deny themselves pleasure. Gambling, workaholism, sex, or even accumulating wealth are some examples. Once you begin the activity, it feels impossible to stop repeating it over and over again.

Reason 2: Overeating in Response to Stress

Do you find yourself reaching for a certain comfort food when you're stressed? For many people, popular comfort foods include a bag of salty potato chips or a pint of their favorite flavor of ice cream. Each crunchy bite of chips or creamy spoonful of ice cream brings them relief from feeling stressed out. Or maybe you stress eat at mealtime, piling your plate with food and consuming every single bite. What's going on here?

First, let's consider what stress is. Stress is a hormonal reaction in your body that makes your heart speed up and tightens your muscles. A stress reaction can be triggered by anything that alters the intensity of your feelings, actions, or communications. It can be brought on by actions or communications that you interpret as being harmful to your safety, security, or health. It might be something as simple as a criticism or negative comment from a co-worker, an argument with a friend, a serious disagreement with your spouse or child, or just excessive worrying about something in your life. Of course, it may also be something that carries with it the threat of actual danger, such as a warning of impending bad weather or being on the freeway with other drivers who are disobeying traffic safety laws and recommendations. Whether the danger ever comes to pass or not, your body gets prepared to deal with it.

The intensity of the trigger leading to a stress response varies for each person. Our conditioning for coping with stress seems to start in early childhood and it continues in adulthood. One individual may be able to manage lots of difficult life events that another person would find highly stressful. What are your stress triggers and how sensitive are you to them?

The hormone adrenaline is released in the body during the stress response. If you remain in a stressful environment or dwell on the stress in your mind, your body continues releasing the hormone for a long period. Adrenaline then brings on the fight-flight-or-freeze response, increasing your heartbeat, tensing your muscles, and deepening your breathing. These responses are meant to help you deal with the stressor.

So how does stress cause people to overeat? If you become stressed when you're hungry, or vice versa, more adrenaline is released. Eating actually helps you feel better because food in your digestive system helps slow the release of adrenaline. However, this experience of feeling calmer after eating can set up a stress-and-eating behavior pattern.

> **If you become stressed when you're hungry, or vice versa, more adrenaline is released. Eating actually helps you feel better because food in your digestive system helps slow the release of adrenaline. However, this experience of feeling calmer after eating can set up a stress-and-eating behavior pattern.**

Here's a second reason people eat when feeling stressed. The body's stress response prompts you to take action to deal with the stressor. For many people, the activity of preparing a meal and eating it helps them stop thinking about the stressor, so they believe they are actually managing the stress. Through the repetition of this behavior, eating can become an automatic coping process for stressed-out people.

DO YOU SEEK AN ADRENALINE RUSH?

The irony about stress is that some people enjoy creating a sense of stress out of ordinary life events. They get used to the adrenaline in their body. They heighten events through thoughts that make them feel internally stressed, and then they believe they become more energetic. In their way of thinking, stress is good for sharpening their focus and performing at a higher level. Some people also utilize stress in a creative way to accomplish their artistic objectives. Others may invent a stressful situation just to experience a thrill, such as driving at high speeds. Do you enjoy an adrenaline rush?

Some folks use food or drink to complement their love of stress. They may drink coffee, soda, and sweetened beverages frequently during the day. In their jobs, they may drive themselves to keep working right through lunchtime, scarfing down snacks and carbohydrate-rich foods and guzzling soda to hold them over until dinnertime.

In the evening, with their body depleted of energy, they finally eat a full meal. However, their lack of balance and control during the day often drives them to overeat at dinner. It has become their only opportunity to enjoy food—and so they overindulge out of the sheer pleasure of tasting the food.

Think about this description of the common behavior pattern of people who enjoy an adrenaline high. Is this you?

Reason 3: Eating Only When You Are Hungry . . . but Overeating

Are you good at waiting for your hunger signals and not eating before that? That's great—but have you noticed that, paradoxically, you seem to be unaware of your body's signals of satisfaction? When you're clueless about being satisfied or full, it's easy to frequently overeat, leading to weight gain. What might cause that? Here are several possible explanations of this behavior.

First, you might overeat because you consume too much of the wrong foods, foods that cause you to put on pounds. For example, your diet may include a lot of grain-based carbohydrates, natural sugars, salt, and fat. While you may believe you are eating appropriate portions, these foods can provide your body with more nutrients than it can immediately use. The skewed choice of foods can fill your body with glucose, fatty acids, and salt. The more you eat these foods, the harder it becomes to maintain your authentic weight and prevent such conditions as high blood sugar and possibly even diabetes.

This type of overeating can begin unconsciously. Although hunger triggers the conscious decision to initiate eating, your subconscious mind is not controlled by rational thought, and it is easily swayed to follow the same eating patterns you established long ago. If you routinely had a big breakfast of eggs, bacon, potatoes, and cinnamon rolls when you grew up, you would likely have a craving for these foods every morning in your adulthood. In effect, you may be hungry when you eat, but you consume too much of the wrong foods out of an embedded habit.

A second reason you may overeat when hungry is that you have delayed eating too long during the day, as do many overworked people who skip lunch. As I pointed out in the sidebar about people who are addicted to an adrenaline rush, when they come home in the evening, their body is depleted of energy by the time they can finally eat a full meal. They are starving and driven to overeat at dinner, because it is their first opportunity to enjoy food in a calm environment that day.

A third reason you may overeat is similar to that of a person who enjoys food and has pleasure-based eating habits. You may wait for the hunger signal, but once it starts, your enjoyment takes over and you cannot stop yourself. The enjoyment itself can even change; instead of eating for variety or quality, the *quantity* of food becomes the pleasure-generating factor for you. It diverts you from paying attention to the feeling of satiation during a meal. Instead, you eat until you feel your stomach literally stretching out—even to the point of discomfort—before you stop eating.

Repeated overeating reinforces the feelings of pleasure you derive from getting full or stuffing yourself, and those feelings become ingrained in your subconscious mind.

This uncontrolled enjoyment may also have started inadvertently by overeating at family events, parties, business outings, and trips where abundant foods are available, often at no monetary cost. Repeated overeating at such times reinforces the feelings of pleasure you derive from getting full or stuffing yourself, and those feelings become ingrained in your subconscious mind.

When you are in your teens or early twenties, the fact that you experience few immediate negative consequences after an excessive intake of food often leads to this overeating behavior pattern. You begin to rationalize overeating with excuses. *I was really hungry. I loved the taste of that new dish.* Or: *I skipped lunch so it's okay if I eat a lot at this party.* You might also be influenced to consume a lot of food by external factors, such as dining at an expensive restaurant where a number of elements are in play, among them enjoyment of the extravagance, concern about getting your money's worth, or other motivations.

Reason 4: Overeating Due to Being Distracted

Distractions while eating can easily lead to overeating. One of the worst culprits is television. Believe it or not, increased food consumption while watching TV has been identified as one of the key contributors to obesity. Why might that be?

When you watch TV while eating, your brain is receiving thousands of messages every second. As the images change on the TV, your brain is constantly shifting its orientation from the signals coming from the taste sensors in your mouth to the rapidly changing sights and sounds on the screen. Out of all those multiple signals, the brain is forced to decide which one gets its primary attention. It might seem like the brain could just decide to focus on food, since that's in your best interest. But did you realize that your brain is programmed to receive messages most strongly through your eyes? In other words, the TV wins and what goes into your mouth loses.

When you watch TV while eating, your brain is receiving thousands of messages every second. When the mind pays no attention to what you're tasting, it's as if you have not tasted it. The quantity of food you consume is thus easy to overlook, and so you just keep eating.

When the mind pays no attention to what you're tasting, it's as if you have not tasted it. The quantity of food you consume is thus easy to overlook, and so you just keep eating. Repeated episodes of eating combined with visual distractions such as the TV can make overeating a regular behavior. The antidote to this behavior is what I call "mindful eating," which you will read about in Chapter 6.

Reason 5: Eating in Response to Clever Food Marketing

This reason for overeating is certainly not news to anyone who lives in the U.S. or any other Western society. We are exposed to an endless barrage of advertising and marketing messages that activate our interest in food and the pleasure of eating. In America, restaurants entice us with daily discounts, special days such as Taco Tuesday, loyalty points, and holiday menus. Many American restaurants, in particular, serve extremely large portions compared to the amount a normal human actually needs for nutrition in a single meal, and their marketing promotes this with visuals of plates piled high. Some restaurants offer "all you can eat" buffets, as if to challenge you to overeat until you are bloated and sick.

In addition, packaged drinks and food products loaded with carbohydrates, sugar, and salt are cleverly marketed in ways that make us associate them with happiness, sexual prowess, success, and good times. Supermarkets tempt us with aisle after aisle of attractively packaged foods and often feature products with highly caloric, processed ingredients at key shelf locations that manufacturers pay for.

It is easy to be enticed by foods that look great or to succumb to persuasive pitches that appeal to your taste buds. But when your diet begins to consist of the wrong foods you can lose control of your health. By falling prey to clever advertising and marketing, you open yourself up to eating the very foods that will cause you to gain weight.

In short, pay attention to how you respond to such advertising and marketing. Are you losing control of your inherent mechanisms to eat healthily and maintain your weight due to these powerful external forces that are skewing your eating patterns? Keep in mind; the companies behind such persuasive messages are mostly motivated to make a profit, not to keep you healthy.

WEIGHT GAIN FROM MEDICAL CONDITIONS AND MEDICATIONS

There is one more reason some people may overeat. Medical conditions related to the heart, thyroid, kidney, and food intake control center in the brain can cause weight gain, whether from overeating or from the condition itself. Also, some medications often have the side effect of stimulating the appetite. Medications such as steroids, antidepressants, insulin, hormones, contraceptives, and anti-seizure drugs can bring on a change in your metabolic rate and nutrient absorption. They can also cause water retention that adds to your weight.

If you find yourself gaining weight while taking a medication, consult your healthcare provider to get clarification. The good news is that the guidance in this book can still help you moderate unwanted weight gain regardless of your medical condition or any medications you may be taking.

Over-Enjoyment Has Become the Norm

Due to the reasons highlighted in this chapter, as well as other factors, obesity rates are on the rise. According to a 2024 report from the Centers for Disease Control and Prevention (CDC), one in five adult Americans (20%) are obese—but in 23 states, that number is one in three (35%). The CDC also notes that obese people are at risk for various health conditions, including high blood pressure, heart disease, stroke, some cancers, and Type 2 diabetes.[2] According to a study published in *The Lancet,* more than

2. https://www.cdc.gov/media/releases/2024/p0912-adult-obesity

1 billion people in the world have to cope with obesity.[3] A revolutionary approach to educating people about how to avoid overeating can go far in reversing these trends in obesity.

If you intend to beat unwanted weight gain, you need to assess whether you are overeating due to any of the reasons we've covered. Which one(s) did you find true for you? Is your overeating now a consistent behavior pattern at every meal? What are some earlier experiences in your life that may have led to this behavior? And finally, be honest with yourself—are you beginning to experience consequences from overeating, e.g., obvious belly fat, high blood pressure, high blood sugar (pre-diabetes), or full-blown Type 2 diabetes?

Once you begin to recognize when you begin to overeat and become aware of which of the mentioned reasons may be driving you to do so, you have an opportunity to change your behavior. You can stop yourself from having an unnecessary snack or meal, and instead heed your natural inclination to eat only when you're truly hungry.

In Chapter 3, you will discover how to reconnect with your natural mechanisms for detecting your body's signals for hunger and satisfaction. You will see that eating the right amount of food to avoid weight gain and stay healthy is literally built into you!

---

3. https://www.who.int/news/item/01-03-2024-one-in-eight-people-are-now-living-with-obesity

Key Points

- The five behavioral reasons why people override their natural signals and overeat include:
  1. Eating for pure enjoyment, even when not hungry.
  2. Eating to relieve stress and anxiety.
  3. Eating only when hungry—but overeating.
  4. Overeating due to being distracted.
  5. Eating in response to clever food marketing.
- Non-hunger eating often begins as a temporary and occasional accident.
- The over-enjoyment of food may seem like no big deal at first. However, through repetition, it becomes a habit.
- When you habitually overeat, you replace your instinctive need to eat for nutrition with eating for other reasons. This can happen despite negative health consequences for your body.

(3)

PAY ATTENTION TO YOUR SIGNALS FOR HUNGER AND SATIATION

In the previous chapter, we discussed how you might be overeating for any of several reasons. In this chapter we'll discuss how you can learn to eat *only* when you're truly hungry and stop when you're satisfied that you have eaten enough.

To beat unwanted weight gain, you need to start paying more attention to two specific types of signals: those your body sends you when you're hungry, and those you receive when you're full.

If you need to ask what those signals feel like, this clearly means you have lost touch with these natural messages. Your daily habit of eating too frequently and too much has taken control over how your body communicates to tell you when to eat and when to stop.

Or maybe you *do* know what these signals are, and you may really feel them, yet you're not acting on them. Well, it's time to respond to them now. You will not be able to shed pounds unless you stop overeating, so you must start listening to these signals and take them into account.

First, let's look more closely at the hunger signals. Understanding exactly what they are can help you regain control of your tendency to eat too frequently and too much.

What Causes the Sensations of Hunger?

Why do you feel the sensations of hunger—the growling of your stomach, the shakiness, the gnawing feeling that you must get some food immediately? There are several theories that seek to explain the hunger signals, but you'd be surprised to learn that the most common ones are illogical. Only one makes sense, biologically speaking.

Here's one theory that is clearly incorrect: The body is programmed to store a certain amount of fat to draw from for energy. This theory believes that hunger signals are the body's way of telling you there's no more fat available. But if this were true, wouldn't people who gain weight, which is stored as fat, cease to be hungry for days, weeks, or even months?

I suggest that the real cause of hunger actually relates to the fact that our brain is a *nutritional regulatory system.* The brain is so sophisticated, it literally keeps track of our nutritional needs, right down to the cellular level.

Another theory says that hunger signals occur when there's not enough glucose in the bloodstream—since glucose is used to fuel our cells. But if low blood sugar causes hunger, then why do people with diabetes get hungry even when their blood sugar levels are far higher than normal? Even people without diabetes feel hunger when their blood sugar levels are kept artificially high with a glucose drip into their veins.

I suggest that the real cause of hunger actually relates to the fact that our brain is a *nutritional regulatory system.* The brain is so sophisticated, it literally keeps track of our nutritional needs, right down to the cellular level.

Think about it, as this is not far-fetched. The brain knows which cells in your left ring finger got pricked when you accidentally touched a thorn on a rose bush. The brain knows to tell specific muscles in your right hand to coordinate with your eye when you play ping-pong. Likewise, the brain is the command center of your nutrition. It has an enormous capacity to track the level of nutrients in every cell of your body.

All day long your cells are consuming nutrients—proteins, fats, glucose, minerals, and vitamins—to power their activities. I suggest that hunger sensations are generated when the brain detects a critical level of depletion, not just of glucose, but also of key nutrients essential for the normal functioning of your body's cells. This is no different than when the brain detects a deficiency of water in your cells and body fluids, and it then generates the sensation of thirst.

Your Brain Determines Your Selection of Foods

Think about how you eat on a daily basis. Perhaps you will realize that you are, in fact, most often choosing your meals based on conscious choices, or even cravings. Through your hunger signals, your brain is often trying to guide you to the right foods. It has learned which foods will provide you with enough of the missing nutrients your cells need.

Did you ever crave something badly, and once you ate or drank it, you had a clear sensation that your body got what it needed? For instance, have you ever craved orange juice, bananas, cheddar cheese, or red meat? Could your craving mean that your body desperately needed Vitamin C, potassium, calcium, or iron—and your brain knew it? It's evident that food cravings are not random messages from the brain. Instead, they are an alarm telling you that your cells need a specific nutrient.

Consider all those times you've asked yourself, "What should I eat for breakfast this morning?" or "What do I want for lunch / dinner today?" Often an answer pops into your head without any problem. This is your brain telling you what nutrients you need, based on its database of foods and their nutrient composition. These messages are different for each person.

Of course, there are times when your brain is rather non-committal. After all, we may not have a specific craving at every meal; our choice of what to eat happens on a subconscious level. We might waver between fish or chicken, a burger or a sub, a raw salad or steamed cauliflower, or a taco or pizza. For many meals, the brain accepts that any of several food choices will satisfy most of your nutrient needs.

In addition, not every meal will supply all the nutrients your cells need. But after each meal, the brain will seek to correct any unmet needs in subsequent meals if necessary. This is why you will often have a strong craving for a certain food after several days of eating other foods that lack those nutrients.

Paying Attention to Hunger Signals Helps You Lose Weight

The brain's regulatory system for nutrient intake applies to humans of all ages—infants, toddlers, children, teens, and adults. Your brain is the CEO of your nutritional regulatory system in the same way that it is the CEO of every other bodily system that keeps you alive.

One way to stop eating too frequently and/or too much is to wait to eat until you sense that your brain is sending you a real hunger signal. Does your stomach feel truly empty? Are you feeling a loss of energy or mental focus? These are the starting signals of genuine hunger.

One way to stop eating too frequently and/or too much is to wait to eat until you sense that your brain is sending you a real hunger signal. Does your stomach feel truly empty? Are you feeling a loss of energy or mental focus? These are the starting signals of genuine hunger. Note they may occur before you experience an actual stomach growl.

As you learn to double-check your awareness of the hunger signals, you may find that you still have a tendency to eat too frequently during the day. I encourage you to review Chapter 2 and ask yourself if you're eating for one of the reasons discussed in that chapter. It can seem normal for you to think you're hungry when you're actually just eating out of stress or to enjoy the pleasure of tasting the food. After all, you've probably developed your overeating habit over many years.

What About the Signals to Stop Eating?

We just explored the hunger sensations—why you become hungry, how your brain guides your selection of foods, and how it tracks your nutritional intake as you eat. Now let's delve into how your brain also informs you when to stop eating during a meal. Paying attention to your satisfaction (also called *satiation*) signals is just as important as being aware of your hunger signals.

The problem is, many people eat until they feel their stomach become completely full. Some people even go beyond that, consuming second and third helpings until they're uncomfortable and full of regret.

So how do you really know when to stop eating?

Once again, it's your brain that literally tells you, but you need to wait long enough for the satiation signals to occur, and then you must pay attention to them. You see, the brain is actually monitoring numerous communications that come from various parts of the body. The brain receives messages from the mouth, the stomach, the intestines, and the blood (see sidebar on the next page)—all of which combine to help it assess when enough nutrients have been consumed to satisfy the demand for nutrition from the body's cells.

How do you really know when to stop eating? Once again, it's your brain that literally tells you, but you need to wait long enough for the satiation signals to occur, and then you must pay attention to them.

Like hunger, satiation signals are highly dependent on your nutritional status. At some meals, you'll need to consume a large quantity before you take in the needed nutrients. At other times, your brain will be satiated even after just a small amount—perhaps because you required a lesser quantity of nutrients, or the food was very rich in the necessary substances.

The tricky thing is that it can take from about 10 or 15 minutes to as many as 30 for the communications from the mouth, stomach, intestines, and blood to combine effectively enough to trigger the brain into sending you the message that says, "Stop eating, you're full." This time lag creates an "overeating danger zone" for you. During those minutes, you probably continue eating out of habit, since your stomach doesn't yet feel as full as you're accustomed to feeling before you stop eating.

SIGNALS FROM THE STOMACH, INTESTINES, AND BLOOD TO THE BRAIN

Your stomach, intestines, and blood (along with your mouth) all offer input that the brain analyzes to determine satisfaction. I'll get to discussing signals from the mouth in the next section; for now, here are some details on the other three. Let's follow the path of your food after it leaves your mouth.

Stomach: As you are aware, chewed food descends down through your esophagus and enters your stomach. The walls of the stomach normally have relatively little muscle tone; this allows the organ to expand and bulge outward as more food enters. At some point the stomach relays to the brain the sensation of being physically full. The problem is, even after eating a huge meal many adults can still find room for more. Their stomach simply expands.

Intestine: From the stomach, food enters the small intestine, where hormones are released. Some of the hormones reach the brain through the blood, informing it that nutrients in the intestine will soon be absorbed. After receiving this information, the brain begins to reduce the intensity of hunger. An interesting aside is that fat-containing foods, such as nuts, speed the release of intestinal hormones faster than carbohydrate foods. This means that your hunger subsides more quickly when eating foods delivering fat. If you're hungry for a snack, it's better to eat nuts than to chomp on some corn chips.

Bloodstream: After digestion begins in the intestines, nutrients such as glucose are released and absorbed into the bloodstream. Blood circulating to the brain lets it know that you've responded to the feeling of hunger, prompting the brain to produce a sense of satisfaction and well-being.

The Key Role of Chewing in Knowing When to Stop Eating

As you read above, it can take time—as much as 30 minutes after you start eating—for messages from the stomach, intestines, and blood to combine in the brain, which then shouts out, *Stop eating!* With this time lag, you might be wondering how it is possible to avoid overeating.

Believe it or not, nature has provided a very clear clue about when to stop eating that you probably have never noticed—and it takes place in your mouth. The taste buds and smell receptors in your mouth play a significant role not only in eating enjoyment, but also in warning you to stop eating.

When you're hungry, the very first bites of food always taste delicious, giving you a powerful sense of enjoyment. As you chew, your teeth break the food up into smaller particles, the molecules of which delight the taste buds, which tell the brain what nutrients are in that food. Similarly, the smell receptors, using chemical sensing, receive molecules and send messages to the brain about the nutritional content of the food.

This is why the parental lecture to "chew your food" is more significant than you might have considered in the past. The more you chew your food, the smaller the particles your teeth will create. The smaller the particles, the more the food releases the molecules of nutrients that your taste buds and smell receptors use to assess the content of the food and communicate it to the brain.

But even more important, chewing plays a key role in helping you know when to stop eating. Here's how.

Have you ever noticed that as you eat, your sense of enjoyment in chewing the food starts to wane little by little? At a certain point, each new bite of food you take no longer produces the same degree of enjoyment as the first bite. The flavors of the food become less distinctive and pleasurable. You may even stop chewing the food as much, just swallowing it in larger chunks as you seek to fill your stomach.

Have you ever noticed that as you eat, your sense of enjoyment in chewing the food starts to wane little by little? The flavors of the food become less distinctive and pleasurable. This loss of enjoyment is nature's first (and major) way of letting you know that you have eaten enough.

This loss of enjoyment is actually nature's first (and major) way of letting you know that you have consumed enough food to derive the necessary nutrients at this time. If you pay close attention to the decrease in your enjoyment, it's a clear tip-off that you're approaching or have even reached the right moment to stop eating.

Once you begin to notice the loss of enjoyment, the best action to take is to stop eating for 10 or 15 minutes.

You can sip on whatever drink you're having. Meanwhile, your brain is collecting the signals from the stomach, intestine, and bloodstream. If you have indeed eaten enough, your brain will send you this additional satiation signal, confirming that you should bring the meal to a close.

Perhaps you're wondering why the process of satiation is so complex? Why do we have so many different inputs for the brain to determine that we should stop eating?

My view is that we developed multiple inputs because many internal and external circumstances can affect our nutritional needs. On some days, the body may need to override the signals from the mouth's taste sensors and smell receptors if the brain determines that not enough of some nutrients have been consumed. Your brain may tell you to keep eating to gain more of some nutrients, even at the risk of overconsuming others.

From a biological point of view, this backup system of four kinds of messages appears to help our survival better than having just one system. If your brain told you to stop eating when you had enough of just one type of nutrient, or a few, you'd never fulfill your body's needs for many types of nutrients.

Putting This Step to Use in Your Life

The human body is a complex organism that survives on its intake of nutrients for energy and the manufacture of various substances it needs. The body has multiple monitoring systems that communicate with the brain so it can tell you when you're hungry and when you have eaten enough. Paying attention to the hunger and satiation signals is a vital

TRUE OR FALSE: I HAVE TO EAT A LOT BECAUSE I HAVE A HIGH METABOLISM.

Some people believe they have a "high metabolism" and therefore have to eat often and a lot, despite the fact that they might be gaining weight. This is a mistaken notion, however. Let me explain.

There are two different meanings of the term *metabolism.* The first refers to the amount of energy your body gets out of each ounce of food; this is your *efficiency of energy extraction.* Each person is different in this sense of the word. Some people are more efficient than others in converting the potential energy in each ounce of food into usable energy. This is like the differences in the efficiency of solar panels made of different materials to convert sunlight to electricity, which can range from 15–23%. Whatever your efficiency, it does not significantly change as you age. However, a person with a *more efficient metabolism* in terms of needing less food energy to do their work risks gaining weight if they consume more food than they need for their energy.

The second meaning of metabolism refers to the total amount of energy you need to use on any given day. This sense of metabolism depends on your body type (i.e., how much muscle mass you have) and the energy needs of your brain and organs. For example, let's say two people each consume 2500 calories per day and do the exact same actions during that day. Each person is different, however, in how many of those calories they need to use. One individual may use 2200 while the other needs only 1800 because of their different body types. Here too, the person who needs to use fewer calories each day may gain weight if they consume more calories than they use.

Meanwhile, a person eating to satisfaction but not gaining weight has a metabolism that is able to use all the calories they consume. Their metabolism is balanced.

Finally, someone who is eating a lot of food but *losing* weight is the person with a high metabolism. Beware, however: this situation can be an indication of a health problem such as hyperthyroidism. They should be sure to consult their medical provider if they fall into this category.

Regardless of your metabolism in *using* food energy, everyone is subjected to nature's will when it comes to aging. What I mean is that the amount of work you can do and the use of energy for that work inevitably decreases as you get older. This is because wear and tear results in loss of muscle volume and strength as you age and you can't generate as much muscle power as you used to have when you were younger.

The point is, you must regulate your food intake as you age and your energy expenditure reduces. Without a corresponding reduction in food intake, you will likely gain weight. Think of it this way: If you use 100 fewer calories per day while consuming the same amount of calories as before, you might gain 10 pounds of weight a year. To prevent weight gain, you need to increase your caloric expenditure through exercise. However, the level of activity necessary to succeed at that is extremely difficult to achieve, if not impossible, especially when you have less muscle mass as you age.

The good news is that becoming overweight is largely preventable by achieving an energy balance between calories consumed and calories used. For most people over age 35, weight gain is due to fat deposits or water retention. The best way to deal with this is to check your weight daily and if it is higher than expected, make adjustments so that you eat a little less during each meal until you lose the excess.

step in learning how to avoid weight gain. It can help you change your unhealthy overeating behaviors.

The next time you think you're hungry, be sure to ask yourself if your desire to eat is truly a response to the hunger signal. If you determine that it is, prepare your food or go out to the restaurant of your choice. However, try this test. Serve yourself the amount of food you normally have, but then eat slowly for about 10 minutes. Chew each bite of food as much as you can before swallowing it. When you have eaten about two-thirds of the food, stop for a few minutes or so. Drink some water to cleanse your mouth.

The next time you think you're hungry, be sure to ask yourself if your desire to eat is truly a response to the hunger signal.

Then start eating again, slowly. Ask yourself if you're still enjoying each bite of food. Have the flavors subsided? Does it taste as good as the first bites? If it does, you may continue to eat until you sense that loss of enjoyment.

Once that happens, stop eating and wait again. See if indeed your brain informs you that your stomach is full and you feel satisfied enough to stop eating. Once you begin to recognize and feel all these satiation signals, you're well on the way to regaining control of your overeating habits.

Key Points

- Hunger signals from your brain guide you toward foods that will deliver the nutrients your body needs.
- Chew your food well to release the molecules so your taste buds and smell receptors can relay the nutritional content in the food to your brain's nutritional monitoring system.
- To determine whether you have eaten enough to satisfy your nutrient needs, your brain assesses four types of messages: signals from your mouth, stomach, intestines, and blood.
- Pay close attention to the intensity of the enjoyment you derive from each bite of food you eat. When the enjoyment decreases, it's the first sign that you're approaching the point at which you should stop eating. Then pay attention to your brain telling you that you have eaten enough and your sense of hunger is satisfied.

(4)

BREAK YOUR OLD EATING AND FOOD-SHOPPING HABITS

Is it really possible to gain control of your unhealthy eating habits? Particularly at those times when you couldn't stop yourself from buying and eating the wrong foods? Fortunately, I have good news for you—*yes, you can!*

You may be thinking, *Of course, it's easy to stop myself. I could do it at any time.* If that were true, then why haven't you done it already?

It's more likely that you're telling yourself the opposite: *I just can't stop myself from indulging in the foods I love. I don't see how I can change my eating habits.* Perhaps this makes you feel skeptical about trying the approach in this book. Perhaps you have experienced failure after failure in the past and are not convinced you can change your lifestyle.

Whatever your reaction, I want to help you feel confident that you *can* regain control. This chapter will introduce you to another approach to beat unwanted weight gain.

The Brain Keeps Track of Your Eating Habits

In the previous chapter, I talked about how your brain keeps track of the nutritional needs of your cells and assesses what nutrients enter your mouth each time you eat. Given this, it shouldn't surprise you that your brain is also ultimately responsible for your eating habits. Starting in childhood, your brain began to track the patterns of your eating habits. Your food experiences produced specific connections between nerve cells in your brain, forming pathways called neural networks.

Over time, the foods and times of day you've been eating have effectively been "hardwired" and solidified into clear neural networks in your brain. These networks are continuously strengthened through years of repeated patterns. They become self-sustaining and, more importantly, very difficult to change; you can't simply delete a neural network like you would a file folder on your computer.

There are good reasons why the brain depends on neural networks. Without well-established transmission channels among nerve cells, critical functions such as heartbeat and respiration might fail—with life-ending results. Another reason the brain forms neural networks is to conserve its energy by being able to make faster decisions. By accessing a pre-formed pathway, the brain saves both time and energy since it doesn't need to test multiple choices.

As you can see, the brain's natural inclination is to form and adhere to neural pathways for many bodily functions. Therefore, it makes sense that it resists any attempt to change a single grouping of connected nerve cells. Trying to consciously modify a pre-formed pathway is actually viewed by the brain as a threat. If an established pathway could easily be altered, even newly formed nerve connections might be overwritten—making it difficult to establish reliable behavior patterns for new situations.

So, Is it Hopeless to Try and Change?

Scientists used to believe that the brain established most of its neural connections during a person's childhood, and that afterward these networks seldom changed. However, research has shown that the brain is far more malleable, with a greater ability to rewire itself than previously assumed. The brain can actually form new connections among different neurons to deal with new situations. Perhaps this is a result of our evolution, where human beings must deal with increasingly complex lives!

Learning that the brain is capable of adapting is very welcome news for anyone wishing to beat unwanted weight gain. You can tap into its resourcefulness to overcome many types of unwanted behaviors and create new outcomes, including better eating habits.

That the brain is capable of adapting is very welcome news for anyone wishing to beat unwanted weight gain. You can tap into its resourcefulness to overcome many types of unwanted behaviors and create new outcomes, including better eating habits. There are two processes that your brain needs to do to accomplish this: unlearning and learning anew. Unlearning requires you to weaken established connections between neurons. Because this work has to be done piecemeal, it takes time. However, it absolutely can be done.

You see, the brain has a natural mechanism that helps you both unlearn old habits and learn new behaviors—using the hormone *oxytocin*. This potent hormone has the power to dissolve existing neural connections so that new ones can be formed. Without this hormone the brain would become saturated with old pathways—leaving no room for new networks or new behaviors to form.

Luckily, the adult brain is fairly accustomed to unlearning and learning anew. If you ever relocated to a new city to study or work, you had to learn how to get around and adjust some of your former habits. Such unlearning of the old and learning of something new required you to "de-connect" established neural paths and make fresh ones. Science refers to this process as *neuroplasticity*—the ability of your brain to alter its neural pathways.

My point is, somewhere in almost everyone's past, they have already unlearned some things and learned new ones. Well, changing your eating habits is no different. I suggest that you can unlearn and learn anew when it comes to your eating behaviors. The same neuroplasticity can help in retraining yourself about how and what you eat.

Unraveling Your Established Pathways Related to Food and Grocery Shopping

To be frank, changing behaviors is not easy. We all have experienced the frustration of trying to change a behavior we don't like. This is because the brain dislikes the uncertainty of new experiences and prefers sticking with what it already knows. To our ancient ancestors, change could mean danger. Faced with the sense that an encounter with new learning is ahead and that it will need to form new pathways, the brain has a way of hesitating. But armed with the right tools, you can overcome your brain's reluctance and make changes happen.

Establishing new behavior patterns that promote healthy eating involves two parts: (1) finding ways to unravel the established pathways and (2) building new neural networks to promote better approaches to eating. Here are my recommendations that will help you with the unlearning phase.

- *Look around your home to identify the sights that test and break your control over food—and eliminate or modify them.* For example, put all food in cabinets where it can't be seen. Don't leave boxes of cookies or doughnuts on your kitchen counters.
- *Work on creating a home environment that is not focused on food.* It's hard to deny the impulse to indulge when you're surrounded by so many pleasing sensations that are commonly paired with eating. Example: If your kitchen table is the place where you, your family, and your friends tend to hang out, move everyone into the living room or patio when possible.
- *Don't shop for groceries on an empty stomach.* Buy food only using a prepared shopping list so you're not tempted to pick up extra items on impulse. For many people, those extra items tend to be packaged foods high in carbohydrates and salt; once they are in your home, it's going to be hard for you to resist eating unhealthy weight-gaining foods.

- *Pre-plan your meals.* Learn about proper portion sizes (see the information in the sidebar on the next page).
- *Avoid locations where you are likely to eat too much or eat the wrong foods.* For you, this may include fast-food establishments, convenience stores and vending machines that prompt you to buy food on impulse, and restaurants with "happy hours" offering low-cost, high-calorie appetizers and drinks.
- *Stop buying or preparing foods you don't want to be eating.* For instance, the sight and smell of sweets like cookies, ice cream, and cakes can stimulate the urge to eat. If these foods aren't in the house, the extra effort of going out to buy them gives you time to reconsider that food choice.

The goal is to decrease temptations you put in front of yourself by reducing the sights, sounds, and smells that trigger your impulses to eat for pleasure.

Creating a Plan to Reduce Stress Eating

A second element of changing your brain's neural networks is to reflect on how much you turn to food for comfort to reduce stress. If your eating behavior is governed by stress, it's time to begin adjusting this response to tension-triggering events. As a stress eater, you have developed many well-established neural pathways in your brain that connect food to calming your anxiety.

If you feel tense often, it may be worthwhile to get professional help with stress management. To help yourself, here are some suggestions for starting to address your stress level and thereby reduce the use of food as a de-stressor.

- *Stop thinking about stressful events.* Do you ruminate about possible future events in a way that stresses you out? One stress-busting step is to minimize the amount of time you spend thinking about or discussing stressful events, particularly those that don't personally concern you. For example, cut back on your consumption

DETERMINING THE RIGHT PORTION SIZE

Frankly, it's impossible for me, or anyone, to tell you the right portion size for you. How much you should eat changes each day, based on your nutrient and energy needs. However, there is an approach I recommend, namely to notice how much you're eating at each meal before you receive the signal of decreased enjoyment. Then figure out your average amounts for different foods. Over time, you'll learn how much you should serve yourself for each type of meal you buy or prepare.

By the way, beware of portion sizes in restaurants. At your favorite restaurant, the portions designated as "small" might conform to the concept of moderation. But keep in mind that every restaurant can and does differ in the size of its portions. In addition, restaurants can simply rename their portion sizes (and change prices) to make customers believe they're eating moderately. Worse yet, many restaurants simply change the appearance of their servings to make unhealthy food look healthier, or they re-label old recipes with a healthy name to fool customers.

One trick to use in restaurants is to share plates with your spouse, significant other, or friends. One of you might order a meat or fish dish while the other orders a salad entrée. I think you may be surprised how satisfied you are with just eating half of each of these dishes. (Or maybe even less!)

of news and social media. Remind yourself that there are still many positive things happening in the world. If somebody is talking to you about their problems, you can feel sympathy and even show compassion by helping them if they ask you to, but avoid getting emotionally involved in their situation.

- *Don't project negative outcomes of your health issues.* Are you coping with an injury or illness? Reduce the stress of the experience by not allowing your imagination to run wild about adverse outcomes. Instead, think about the ways you can help yourself recover and note your progress. Even if complications do occur, they may not be as severe as you might imagine.
- *Don't project unfavorable outcomes of events in your own life.* Limit your expectations to strictly what you have full knowledge of. Otherwise, developing worried feelings related to future outcomes could become progressively more depressing. You could be filling your mind with anxious thoughts that trigger the release of stress hormones and lead you to reach for food to feel better. Each time your thoughts go negative, your brain recruits more neurons for that gloomy path. This dark train of thought also solidifies the neural connections, intensifying your stress. For relief, take active steps to move your thinking in a positive direction. Meditation is one possible method to do that.

By taking these steps to reduce your stress load, you'll feel less anxiety and decrease your emotional reactivity. This can go a long way to curbing your stress eating.

LESSEN YOUR STRESS WITH MEDITATION

There's a well-proven method to reduce the impact of stress: meditation. One of the reasons meditation seems difficult is precisely because brain neurons are programmed to respond to signals from outside the body, from internal parts of the body, and from other neurons. Meditation calms the brain by asking you to quiet the mind and stop all signal processing.

Meditation is useful for people seeking to retrain their stress responses. With practice, it can build a new network of neurons that avoid all incoming signals, thus creating an environment of peace and calm. Eliciting this string of neurons during meditation is a welcome escape for the mind. It allows those neurons that have been dealing with the stress to rest and recuperate. By processing the stress response from a new perspective, you also may tap into a different set of neurons.

I have created a simple meditation that anyone can do. Use the QR code to go to the online page where I teach you how to perform this meditation.

Tapping into Your Willpower

As you begin changing your patterns of eating—such as why you eat, what you eat, and, more importantly, how you eat—one of the most significant steps you can take is to tap into your willpower. What does this mean?

We commonly call the self-control to resist something negative or to do something positive with regard to improving our lives *willpower.* You need willpower to resist eating when you're not hungry and to eat only when you are hungry, as we discussed in Chapter 3. You also need self-control to stick with eating the right foods in the right portion sizes.

So how do you tap into your willpower? Effectively, your willpower is a function of how you talk to yourself and then how you act in response to that self-talk. Willpower is your inner voice that tells you to remember your commitment to beat weight gain. Without it, you're bound to come up with excuses for why you can eat a second helping or an unhealthy, calorie-packed snack.

Your willpower is a function of how you talk to yourself and then how you act in response to that self-talk. Willpower is your inner voice that tells you to remember your commitment to beat weight gain. Without it, you're bound to come up with excuses for why you can eat a second helping or an unhealthy, calorie-packed snack.

Of course, you don't always have control over the sights, sounds, and smells that can trigger your desire to eat, especially in places outside of your own environment. But you can moderate the effect of these cues by changing what happens in your brain when these sensory impulses are received. For this, your self-talk has to decide consciously to override your longtime conditioned responses.

For example, you literally have to be able to tell yourself to resist the many temptations that cross your path. This can include the aroma of bread or cookies baking at the mall, the sound of bacon or sausages sizzling at the diner where you get your coffee, or the sight of a co-worker's birthday cake in the break room. Know that exposure to any of these food cues doesn't mean it's okay to eat if you're not hungry. Instead, tap into your willpower.

Your supportive thoughts coming to you through your inner voice are the manifestation of that willpower. With effort and training, you can hush the voice of temptation and keep your focus on better choices.

It's helpful to keep in mind two important incentives when you talk to yourself about food. Apply these to your self-talk the next time you're tempted to eat when you're not hungry, or you've already eaten enough and are approaching overeating. The first of these is: *If I can train myself to eat better, I will stay healthier longer.* The second is: *I will feel and look better and enjoy life far more by maintaining my authentic weight.*

Be aware that tapping into your willpower needs to become a conscious response for you whenever you're tempted by food. And it should also remain top of mind. It's hard to exercise your willpower if your thinking is preoccupied with other pressing matters. Make sure your willpower is given as much importance as any other important factors in your life.

Reflect on Your Childhood Eating Habits

I wrote earlier that your childhood eating habits were based on true hunger and satisfaction, especially in infancy. You ate enough to grow and function, but you didn't overeat. Over time, however, your parents, other people, the cultural environment in which you lived, the choices presented to you, and your life experiences all contributed to modifying, if not corrupting, your healthier childhood eating patterns.

YOU ALREADY HAVE WILLPOWER

As a positive reminder that you *can* tap into your willpower, think about another area of life where you're successful in benefiting from willpower. For instance, if you get to your job every morning on time, you have willpower. If you pay your mortgage payment or rent on time each month, you have willpower. If you clean your house every Saturday without fail, you have willpower. You already have willpower, and you can apply it to your eating habits as well.

In what areas of your life do you already demonstrate willpower? Write them down and use the same self-talk on your eating habits that you use for those other habits, tasks, or activities.

Your mission now is to rediscover your authentic weight and learn to eat to maintain it. You can give yourself a psychological boost if you recall your early childhood, when you probably didn't worry about your weight. I suggest that you think of your journey to beat weight gain as reestablishing the eating behavior of your early childhood days, behavior that matched your body's need for nutrients. This goal can help you internalize the thought that if your need for nutrients is not real, you shouldn't be eating.

Don't Be Swayed by Advertising or Social Situations

In our modern world, we're surrounded by marketing and advertising messages that directly and indirectly involve food. Print, TV, and social media ads intentionally seek to create in their audiences the urge to eat. Your exquisitely trained brain, instead of responding to nutrient needs, is tempted many times per hour to imagine the pleasure of eating the foods in the ads.

You need to look deeply at what causes you to give in to the temptations related to food. What are your motivations to believe and accept a TV or print advertisement that you know was intentionally created to appeal to, and even create, your unhealthy desires? It could be that the advertisement presents some new type of food that you want to try out of curiosity. Or the motivation could be deeper than that. Perhaps you feel bored from not having enough meaningful things to do in your life, or you get tired from long days at a demanding job, an overcommitted volunteer schedule, or seemingly endless chores and responsibilities at home. In addition, if stress frequently triggers you to eat, could you actually be creating drama in your life in order to get a lift from an anxiety rush?

Given the overwhelming world of advertising, you must recommit every day to adhere to your vision of eating in a healthier way to avoid weight gain. Look at advertising for what it is—a play on your emotions, and not your rational thoughts about a healthy diet. Remember: the advertisers and marketers don't care if you gain weight, become obese, or develop Type 2 diabetes!

Given the overwhelming world of advertising, you must recommit every day to adhere to your vision of eating in a healthier way to avoid weight gain. Look at advertising for what it is—a play on your emotions, and not your rational thoughts about a healthy diet. Remember: The advertisers and marketers don't care if you gain weight, become obese, or develop Type 2 diabetes!

Similarly, when you're out at a restaurant or at somebody's house, you can be tempted again to abandon your commitment. You'll feel that you have less control because your food choices are limited by the menu or what the host is serving. You have to stay alert and use your self-talk as you decide what and how much to eat. Remember to enjoy what you've selected and recall that a reduction in flavor is your cue to stop eating.

HOW OUR CONSCIOUS CHOICES OVERRIDE OUR NEED FOR NUTRIENTS

Nature has programmed us to eat and enjoy food from the day we are born. Consider, for example, how a newborn will consume enough food to achieve tripling of its body weight during just the first year of life. As we grow, we experience changes in our needs for nutrients almost daily, though most changes are slow and imperceptible. In our toddler years, there is a measurable reduction in our need for nutrients and energy compared to the first year of life because of a slower rate of growth and weight gain. It is at this age when most parents complain that their toddler does not eat enough. In our teen years, we undergo a growth spurt as we are building muscle mass and lengthening our bones. As a result, teens usually consume large amounts of food, but do not tend to gain weight because any excess fat is quickly used to produce energy as needed between meals.

As we grow into adults, however, we usually fall into patterns of eating that are highly influenced by our family and our friends' eating behaviors, taste preferences, and culture. In our thirties or forties our energy needs may be reduced and our metabolism may slow down. We begin to gain weight.

Many people justify the extra pounds because they see everyone around them experiencing it.

So, the question is this: If our brain tracks our nutrient needs, why doesn't it stop us from overeating in our adult years? Doesn't the brain know we need fewer nutrients as our energy needs decline? The fact is, there really is no evidence that the brain does lose its ability to track our nutrient needs. We should be able to balance our food intake to match the nutrients needs of our cells.

So what could possibly be the reason for unwanted weight gain? It seems clear that the problem lies at the behavioral level. Our conscious mind is simply overriding the prompts from the subconscious mind telling us how much food we actually need. Our own behavioral choices are behind our many bad habits, such as why we eat when we are not hungry, why we select unhealthy foods, why we consume huge portion sizes to get our money's worth, why we eat fast foods that require little or no chewing, why we eat too fast due to lack of time to enjoy each bite, and why we keep eating until our stomach is full and we feel uncomfortable.

Here's the bottom line: It is up to you to begin saying no to your conscious impulses if you are serious about beating unwanted weight gain.

How to Avoid Falling into Prior Habits

To change your behavior, you'll have to destroy many established nerve connections and form new ones. This will take time. The strength of your brain's existing networks is why it's easy to reactivate old connections and fall back into familiar former patterns. How much importance you give to your new way of eating will determine how effective you are at rewiring your brain. You must not only learn to do things that work, but also avoid falling back into your previous habits.

Here's an analogy that can help you picture what you need to do. Imagine that an orchestra has been performing a particular piece of music for a very long time under a certain conductor. Then a new conductor is hired, and the musicians are asked to perform the music in a different way. This style is similar to the earlier way they had been performing, but with variations in note strength, tempo, and volume. It would be hard for most of the members of the orchestra to avoid falling back to the way they were accustomed to playing the music, unless they really concentrate. Making such a change takes a while to get it right. However, with practice, soon the new piece becomes as hardwired as the previous one, if not more so.

In a similar way, there will be times when you'll find it hard to stick to your commitment to listen to your new conductor (your brain after reading this book). The old neural pathways will keep trying to dictate your behavior. One common instance of this occurs when the neurochemicals needed for exercising self-control are not available. For example, at the end of a long day at work, it's possible your neurons may be depleted of the neurochemicals needed to generate a disciplined behavior. You might find yourself falling back into old habits. Before you know it, you're eating an unhealthy snack, even without the hunger sensation being triggered.

It can take weeks to dismantle old networks and establish new pathways for different behaviors around eating. Even after that initial phase, making the behavior permanent can require months of practice. So you must keep working on it. Repetition not only strengthens the connections between certain populations of neurons, it also makes it easier to activate them. Note that if you reach a plateau in your progress, it's often a sign that your brain needs time to consolidate the changes already made before you can move forward with additional changes.

Establishing a behavior pattern conducive to maintaining your authentic weight requires commitment and determination. Yet once the pattern is firmly established, it becomes relatively easy to follow. By repeating your new behavior day after day, like an orchestra practicing a new way of performing the same piece of music, changes in your brain connections will become more refined and established, and the new behavior more automatic.

Key Points

- Throughout your life, each time you ate something your brain received millions of signals from your taste and smell receptors. Over time, the way you've been eating has effectively been "hardwired" and solidified as a neural network in your brain. This makes changing eating behaviors difficult, but unlearning can be done.
- We now know that the brain has more of an ability to rewire itself than previously assumed. This resourcefulness of the brain can be used to overcome an established unwanted behavior and accomplish a positive new outcome—such as achieving the better eating habits you desire.

- To establish a new behavior pattern that promotes healthy eating, find ways to stop activating the established pathways that promote unhealthy eating. For instance, don't buy or prepare foods you don't want to be eating.
- If your eating behavior is governed by stress, you'll want to adjust your response to stressful events in general—in addition to changing your pattern of eating. This is because your eating response is interconnected with your reactions to stress, and thus runs through the many well-established and linked pathways in your brain.
- Tap into your willpower—your self-talk—to keep reminding yourself of positive messages and overcome your natural resistance to change. Make a list of situations where you have demonstrated willpower. Post the list in a prominent place (on the refrigerator, on your bathroom mirror, on the full-length mirror in your bedroom) to remind yourself that you can do this. Acknowledge your willpower and feel proud of yourself.
- It may take several weeks to modify the neural networks in your brain and delete old connections about eating, but it can be done. If you reach a plateau in your progress, it simply means your brain needs time to consolidate the changes already made, so be patient.

(5)

REDUCE YOUR CONSUMPTION OF GRAIN-BASED CARBS

To lose weight, one of the most impactful changes you can make is to reduce your consumption of grains and grain-flour products. By grains, I am referring to wheat, rye, barley, oats, rice, and corn. All these grains are also used to create a wide range of grain-flour products, including many types of bread, pizza, tacos, doughnuts, muffins, cakes, pies, pastries, and the list goes on. When you start reducing how much of these you eat each day, you will begin shedding pounds. This simple change in your diet can help you lose one pound per week.

Why do you need to cut out grain-based carbohydrates? This chapter will explain in simple terms how these complex carbohydrates contribute to weight gain more than any other food you can eat.

Understanding Sugar vs. Glucose as the Cause of Weight Gain

Our love of sweetness must have started eons ago when our hunter-gatherer ancestors consumed berries and fruits, and they found the taste enjoyable. As babies, our first taste of food is milk, which contains a form of sugar so its flavor includes sweetness. As adults, whenever our taste buds encounter sweetness, this sends signals to the brain that produce a pleasing response. We know that sugar provides energy to cells, but it's likely that your notions about the word *sugar* include some misunderstandings. Here's why.

Many people think that too much of the white or brown table sugar they put in their coffee is a major cause of weight gain. They may also think that too much white or brown table sugar is the culprit behind the "high blood sugar" associated with Type 2 diabetes. Thus, they stop adding sugar to their coffee while eating a nice big muffin. While the added sugar can be a factor in high blood sugar, this change reflects a misunderstanding of what *blood sugar* actually means.

When we talk about blood sugar, we are referring to glucose—the final result of your body digesting and breaking down many of the foods you eat.

Where does glucose come from? Here is a simple explanation. It comes from three different types of natural sugars found in food and digested in your stomach and intestines. This information is truly worth learning and remembering, as it is the foundation of your understanding weight gain as well as whether you might develop high blood sugar and potentially Type 2 diabetes. Here are the three types of sugars from which glucose (blood sugar) is derived:

- *Sucrose* (natural sugar) is found in fruits, berries, sugar cane, sugar beets, and other crops that can be boiled down into granulated sugar or sugar syrup. A molecule of sucrose is made up of equal amounts of glucose and *fructose.* When you eat a piece of fruit, put jam on your toast, or add sugar to your coffee, you are indeed adding some glucose to your bloodstream. But the fructose portion of sucrose molecules is absorbed only half as fast as the glucose portion; also, each fructose molecule has to be modified in the liver to a glucose molecule before it can elevate blood sugar.

- *Lactose* is the form of sugar found in dairy products; these include milk, cheese, cream, yogurt, ice cream, and butter. Like sucrose, a molecule of lactose is a compound, composed of 50% glucose and 50% *galactose.* Each molecule of galactose must be further processed by the liver to glucose before it can elevate your blood sugar.
- *Maltose* is the form of sugar found in complex carbohydrates that are broken down into glucose. The more bread, pasta, rice, and potatoes you eat, the more you fill your bloodstream with pure glucose.

Here is a chart that can help you remember these three types of sugars in food.

NATURAL SUGARS

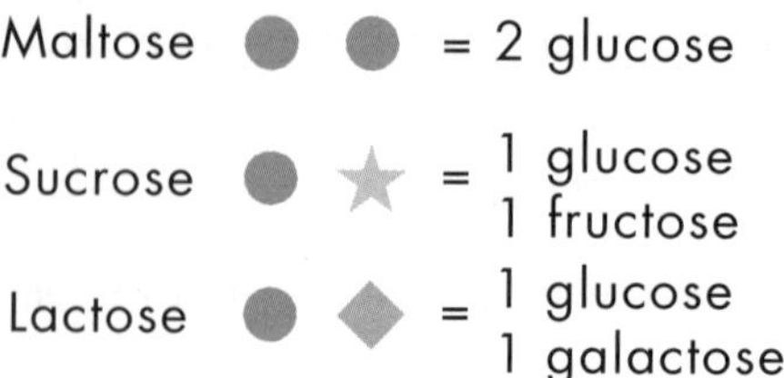

What does learning about these three types of sugar have to do with weight gain? Here is the point:

Most of the glucose you put into your bloodstream that causes weight gain comes from eating complex carbohydrates, not from the sucrose in fruits, or the lactose in dairy products. The more carbohydrates you eat, the greater the chances you will gain weight.

Let's look closer now at why carbohydrates are the main cause of unwanted weight gain.

Weight Gain Enemy #1—Grain-Based Carbohydrates

Before now, you may not have realized that the most substantial filler of your fat cells—which results in your gaining weight—is grain-based carbohydrates. This includes the complex starches—wheat, oats, barley, corn, rice, rye, and others. All of these complex carbohydrates break down into HUGE amounts of glucose in your bloodstream. These carbs introduce far more glucose into the bloodstream than other foods with sugar molecules, such as fruit (delivering sucrose) or milk products (containing lactose). Many vegetables also produce some amount of glucose after digestion, but not nearly as much as grain-based carbohydrates. In short, the more bread, bagels, muffins, doughnuts, pasta, pizza, tortillas, and rice you eat, the more you fill your body with glucose.

Your body does need some carbohydrates. They serve a valuable purpose as one of the body's sources of energy needed to power cells. Glucose from carbohydrates is always present in the bloodstream and in the fluid around the cells.

Muscles use large amounts of glucose during exercise, especially during the early seconds of intense movement.

The problem is this, though: If your meals are constantly high in carbohydrates that result in voluminous amounts of glucose in your bloodstream, your body's cells cannot utilize all of this glucose. A small amount of it is stored in the liver in the form of *glycogen*, to be used between meals when cells may need an extra hit of glucose for energy.

But the majority of glucose in your bloodstream is converted into *triglycerides* (i.e., three fatty acid molecules linked together) that are sent to your fat cells for storage. And, of course, the more you fill your fat cells, the more pounds you gain.

> **How much carbohydrate should you eat? As a general rule, I suggest you keep your consumption of carbohydrates to less than 30% of your total daily caloric intake. Unfortunately, most Americans consume 50% or more of their daily caloric intake in the form of carbohydrates, largely from grains and grain-flour products. That's way too much. This level of carb consumption explains the explosion of overweight people and obesity in the U.S. and in many developed nations of the world.**

The takeaway from this explanation about glucose is this:

If you want to shed pounds and never put them back, reduce the amount of carbohydrates that you consume each day—especially from grains and grain-flour products.

How much carbohydrate should you eat? As a general rule, I suggest you keep your consumption of carbohydrates to less than 30% of your total daily caloric intake. Unfortunately, most Americans consume 50% or more of their daily caloric intake in the form of carbohydrates, largely from grains and grain-flour products. That's way too much. In my view, this level of carb consumption explains the explosion of overweight people and obesity in the U.S. and in many developed nations of the world.

Do you sense this includes you? Do you eat a lot of breads, rolls, tortillas, muffins, doughnuts, pizza, rice, cakes, and other grain-based products every day? If so, you need to make an effort to cut back on your carb consumption. As you learn to better recognize and listen to your hunger and "stop eating" signals, you'll get a sense for how much carbohydrate you should be eating each day.

6 Steps for Cutting Back Carbs

Try out the following six suggestions for just eight weeks, and you'll see that they will likely help you lose weight. Losing just one pound per week can make a real difference in your lifestyle and health.

1. *Avoid muffins, bagels, doughnuts, Danish, and large servings of grain-based cereals for breakfast.* A slice of toast or a small bowl of oatmeal can suffice, along with eggs or breakfast meats if desired.

2. *Skip eating high-carb lunches every day, such as sandwiches, pizza, tacos, rice dishes, pasta, and so on.* A few days per week, substitute a vegetable-based dish, a chef's salad, or a lettuce-wrap sandwich to cut your weekly carb intake.

3. *Reduce the frequency of eating rice, white potatoes, corn, or bread rolls with your lunches and dinners.* If included, reduce the portion size of a serving.

4. *Pay attention to the calories in most fast-food sandwich items.* Many of them exceed 1000 calories or even 1500 calories in a single serving, most of which is from the bread or rolls the meat is served on. One solution to reduce the caloric intake is to eat it as an open-faced sandwich by removing the top slice of bread.

5. *It doesn't matter if you're eating "whole grain" or "gluten-free" bread, cereals, or desserts*; most are still made from grain carbohydrates that digest into glucose. One exception is products made from cauliflower, but many of these also contain rice or potato flour.

6. *Reduce your consumption of high-carbohydrate, high-sugar desserts* such as cookies, cakes, pies, and so on.

5 MORE WAYS TO CUT BACK ON CARBS

Here are five additional ways you can lower your consumption of grain-based carbs.

1. ***Eat nuts or suck on a hard candy when you feel hungry.*** If you crave a morning or afternoon snack and tend to go for a pastry, doughnut, or other high-carb sweet, eating nuts will help you to moderate your hunger longer. If that is not possible, suck on a hard candy containing natural sugar. Though it delivers only a small amount of sugar, the quickness of relief seems to reassure the brain that glucose is on the way. In research tests, just 100 milligrams of sugar reduced the intensity of hunger in subjects.

2. ***Stop eating grains and carbs that don't need to be chewed or require little chewing.*** This includes mashed potatoes, rice, soft breads, and pastries made from grains or corn-based products. Replace these with edible tubers and roots, such as sweet potatoes, yams, and taro. Also, consider lentils as a side dish; the fibers naturally present in lentils take longer to digest, and, therefore, they result in a much slower elevation of blood sugar.
3. ***Chew all your food more slowly.*** Slow chewing helps your brain regulate your digestive process and makes you more aware of the signal to stop eating when you sense the lessening of taste in your mouth.
4. ***Leave an increasing amount of food on your plate.*** If you're overweight, one cause might be that your portion sizes are too large. Seek to adjust them, and remember to chew slowly. Start by leaving 1/8 of the food on your plate, then 2/8 (1/4), and finally up to 1/3 of the food served to you. Of course, the most useful foods to leave on your plate so that you lose weight are the carbohydrates made from grains. By the way, if you are concerned about wasting food when following this training process to eat less, keep in mind that soon you will get used to eating smaller portions and it will become a matter of habit to keep that unnecessary quantity of food off your plate when you first serve it.
5. ***Add herbs and spices to all your dishes.*** Natural herbs and spices are great sources of micronutrients. When you cook using spices, the brain anticipates the arrival of a needed micronutrient in the mouth. That's one reason spices make meals more enjoyable. As you gradually incorporate more herbs and spices into your diet, wean yourself off of grain and grain-flour products.

The Risk of Developing Type 2 Diabetes Due to Excessive Carb Consumption

Let me draw your attention to an important concern you should have about filling your fat cells by overconsuming grains. Did you know that every human being has only a certain amount of fat cells and stem cells that can become fat cells in the body? This amount is determined by your individual genetic makeup. Each member of a family has their own unique combination of genes, half from the mother and half from the father. That explains why one sibling can be tall and skinny, while another is shorter and stockier.

My research on weight gain, obesity, and high blood sugar suggests that at some point, many people effectively fill all their fat cells and stem cells that become fat cells. Once all your fat cells are full, it leaves nowhere for the triglycerides made from the excess glucose in your bloodstream to be stored. These triglycerides are then broken back down into small molecules of fatty acids that flow through the bloodstream.

What happens next is my theory on the cause of Type 2 diabetes, which I call the "fatty acid burn switch." Here's what I mean. We know that muscle cells are like a hybrid car that can use either gasoline or electricity to power the engine. In the same way, muscle cells can burn either glucose or fatty acids. I propose that when fatty acids are flowing through the blood, they enter muscle cells, where they are used to power the cells. As a result, muscle cells do not need the glucose in the bloodstream from the recent meal or from the liver. The consequence is that the glucose remains in the bloodstream, thus high blood sugar.

There is great danger in having consistently high blood sugar over a long period of time. You can develop Type 2 diabetes. I mention this danger many times in this book because this condition is not to be minimized; it leads to many health complications.

In Type 2 diabetes, the voluminous numbers of glucose molecules in your bloodstream become attached to different proteins, a process called *glycation.* The body can tolerate a certain amount of glycation without ill effects. However, too much of it over long periods of time can lead to impairment of cell functions in organs, nerves, and the brain. Glycation can cause nerve damage in the legs and feet, leading to limb amputation. It can damage nerves in the eyes, causing blindness. It is also commonly accepted by researchers that Alzheimer's disease starts with glycation of proteins in the brain.

There is great danger in having consistently high blood sugar over a long period of time. You can develop Type 2 diabetes. This condition is not to be minimized; it leads to many health complications.

It's Not Fat that Makes You Fat

As you have read in this chapter, overconsuming carbohydrates from grains is the major cause of weight gain. Putting on pounds is due to an excessive amount of glucose in your bloodstream that, if not used immediately, are converted to triglycerides that are stored in your fat cells. Little by little, you increase your fat cell storage—and you gain weight!

The primary role of carbs in weight gain may be shocking news to you. Many people have long believed that consuming foods containing fat is what makes them fat. They thus eat a low-fat diet, avoiding fatty meats, oils, cheese, other dairy products, and so on.

The problem is, a low-fat diet often results in people eating a lot of carbohydrates to fill their stomach. They overconsume bread, pizza (without cheese), rice, and other grains. Here's how this misconception came about.

In the 1960s, an experiment was conducted to ascertain the role of fats in causing heart disease and arteriosclerosis. The results inaccurately led Americans to believe that fats were the worst foods to eat and could lead to premature heart attack, stroke, and death. As a result of misleading research, doctors, nutritionists, and food gurus everywhere started promoting diets low in fat. Since then, people have begun substituting carbohydrates in their diets to replace the lost calories from fats. Today, more than fifty percent of the food calories in an average adult's diet is made up of carbs.

The nature of what creates fat in your body is misunderstood. The majority of the fat that fills your fat cells doesn't come from the lipids in meat and dairy. Most of it derives from the glucose you consume in carbohydrates.

Over time, some of the research on the linkage between fat and heart disease has been disproven. New research is furthering our knowledge that not all fat is bad. In recent years, other research has shown that even saturated fats may not be as bad for the body as they have been made out to be.

In short, the nature of what creates fat in your body is misunderstood. The majority of the fat that fills your fat cells doesn't come from the lipids in meat and dairy. Yes, it is true that fats break down into saturated and unsaturated fatty acids, some of which are transformed into triglycerides that end up also filling your fat cells. But most of the fat in your fat cells derives from the glucose you consume in carbohydrates.

The bottom line: It is the overconsumption of carbs in our everyday diet that we must rethink.

The case against dietary fat must be reevaluated. A significant proof against the low-fat diet is that it has led directly to an explosion of obesity and diabetes in the U.S. The scientific community has had a major epiphany, recognizing that carbohydrates, not fats, present the greatest danger to our health.

So, the case against fat is beginning to crumble, and scientists no longer view fats as the worst offender in causing disease and mortality. If you have been following a low-fat diet, consider reevaluating your basis for doing so. I'm not suggesting that you eat as much fatty meat and dairy as you wish. Instead, I am proposing that you always eat what you enjoy, letting your brain guide you to the necessary nutrients. But at the same time, pay attention to your portion sizes, your consumption of grains and grain-flour foods, and to your body's hunger and "stop eating" signals so that you can avoid overeating on an everyday basis.

Remember this:

Nature never intended for human beings to consume so much carbohydrate that we'd create the conditions for weight gain and Type 2 diabetes by filling up our fat cells.

WHY DOES OUR BODY STORE FAT?

Here's a little science for those interested in going deeper. Fat is the body's preferred method of storing energy nutrients that aren't put to immediate use. But how did this come about? There are various theories.

One leading theory proposes that our evolutionary ancestors had to develop some capacity to store energy in the form of fat because they faced periods of famine. The genes responsible for creating fat cells to store energy were seen as a survival advantage. But I suggest that because the body cannot survive on stored fat alone, this theory is suspect. The body also needs a proportional amount of protein, carbohydrates, vitamins, minerals, and trace elements. However, these don't have storage locations in the body.

Here's what I believe is the real reason we store fat. It's the best way humans have to ensure we get access to all the nutrients our body needs. In those early days of human evolution, we often had to ingest an excess of food just to get the proteins, vitamins, and minerals we needed to survive. In that process, we ended up overconsuming foods that produced an excess of glucose, which converted to triglycerides and fatty acids. Since the body could not excrete the triglycerides and fatty acids, it created a mechanism to store them—fat cells.

Watch Your Salt Consumption Too

You may not realize this, but too much salt also plays a role in your gaining unwanted weight. Let me explain how this happens. But first, let's take a look at how much salt a person actually needs and then we can define what is too much salt and how it impacts your gaining weight.

For most of human history, people didn't consume much salt because it was not plentiful. In ancient Rome, most salt was dug out of salt mines by prisoners and slaves; this was because the mining work was grueling and dangerous, as breathing salt for long periods of time often led to dehydration and life-threatening respiratory problems. Some civilizations learned to evaporate salt from the ocean. Since mining and making sea salt were expensive and difficult operations, salt was a highly valued commodity throughout most of human history. A luxury that most people could not afford.

The biochemistry of the human body shows that we have a need for a *small amount* of salt in our diets. But what we actually require are the two chemical components of salt—sodium (Na) and chloride (Cl). It doesn't matter if the salt comes from mines or the sea, as both types are chemically the same. (Sea salt may contain other minerals the body can use.)

Sodium contributes to keeping our fluid balance, blood pressure, muscle activity, and electrical signal transmission healthy. At a cellular level, sodium controls water movement in and out of the cells.

So how much salt does a person need? The Food and Drug Administration (FDA) recommends no more than 2300 milligrams daily, but I believe this is still too high. An adequate amount is between 1200 and 1500 milligrams daily. The problem is, most people consume far more salt. Studies confirm that there is an extremely high level of salt consumption among children and adults today. In 2024, the Centers for Disease Control stated that Americans consume 3300 milligrams of salt daily, compared to 2300 milligrams decades ago. That's an extra teaspoon of salt a day. The most sodium you likely consume (as much as 70% of your daily intake, according to the FDA) comes from processed or packaged foods and restaurant foods.

Too much salt plays a role in your gaining unwanted weight, so cut back on your salt intake. Studies have shown that people who consistently limit salt in their diets eventually adapt to eating less salty foods.

Here's how too much salt can affect your ability to lose weight. There's a biological dynamic known as the sodium-carbohydrate interaction. When you digest carbohydrates, a large quantity of glucose is released in the intestine. In order to be absorbed by your cells, that glucose must be dissolved in water. But moving water into cells requires sodium molecules.

So when you eat more carbohydrates, it prompts the brain to desire more sodium to help move the water. This is why you often crave salt or salty accompaniments when you eat breads, pasta, snack foods, and so on. Furthermore, most high carb processed foods in the modern diet are loaded with too much salt. This creates a repetitive negative cycle that can launch you into a weight gain pattern.

But that's not the only problem. Another concern with too much salt in your diet is this: Sodium ions attach to water molecules; too much salt causes your body to hold on to too much water, increasing your blood volume. Significant increases in blood volume can result in elevated blood pressure, which can raise your risk of heart attack, heart failure, stroke, kidney disease, and blindness.

If you want to lose weight, you need to cut back on your salt intake. Studies have shown that people who consistently limit salt in their diets eventually adapt to eating less salty foods. In fact, they can taste it when food is too salty and end up preferring less salty meals.

Seven Ways to Curb Your Salt Intake

Here are some ways to reduce your taste for salty foods:

1. *Cut down on your consumption of carbohydrates.* We live in an environment where nearly every global cuisine has evolved to incorporate more and more complex carbohydrates. Fight the trend. Reducing your intake of carbs is the most important action you can take to prevent the sodium-carbohydrate cycle.

2. *At your meals, stop eating when the food is no longer enjoyable.* This is your brain telling you that your body no longer needs any of the nutrients left. Chew your food slowly and savor the flavors. You'll become more aware of how highly salted many foods are.

3. *When you cook, try gradually decreasing the amount of salt you add.* Cut the salt you add by $^1/_8$, then $^1/_4$, then by $^1/_3$, and finally to the smallest amount of salt possible.

With less salt, you'll find it easier to appreciate the natural flavors of the ingredients of your meals. You can also enhance flavors with herbs and spices.

4. *Pay attention to the sodium content of processed and packaged foods when shopping.* At the grocery store, read the food labels to avoid items containing more than 480 mg. of sodium in one serving. You cannot rely on your taste buds to know if something is salty, because they may be unable to detect how salty some foods are, especially if the salinity of your saliva is higher due to the high salt content of your blood. An easy way to remember how much salt is OK in a canned or packaged product is to make sure the sodium content (in milligrams) is not higher than the calories per serving. For example, if the calories per serving are 100, the sodium content should be 100 milligrams or less per serving.

5. *Avoid buying cured meats and processed foods packaged in ready-to-eat single servings.* These items are likely to contain high levels of salt.

6. *Watch out for canned vegetables and legumes*, as they often contain a lot of salt. After opening a can, rinse the food under cold running water to reduce the salt content by about 40%.

7. *Buy raw nuts that you roast without salt for snacking.* Walnuts roasted in the oven without oil, for example, make an excellent snack food.

All these recommendations can help you in due course to consume very little salt, which will help you control your cravings for carbohydrates. The less salt you eat, the greater your chances of being able to lose weight or control it.

Key Points

- Your sugar consumption is something to stay on top of, especially because the sweet taste is so tempting.
- The biggest single filler of your fat cells is grain-based carbohydrates. These include the complex starch foods of the grain family—wheat, oats, barley, corn, rice, rye, and others—as well as potatoes, all of which break down into glucose. Carbohydrates now account for over 50% of the calories in the typical U.S. diet. That's way too much. Eating excessive amounts of carbs will undermine your effort to beat weight gain.
- The nature of what creates fat in your body is misunderstood. The majority of the fat that fills your fat cells doesn't come from the lipids in meat and dairy. Most of the fat in your fat cells derives from the glucose you consume in carbohydrates. Excess glucose not immediately used after a meal is stored in your fat cells, leading to weight gain.
- While we do need some salt in our diet, studies confirm that there is an extremely high level of salt consumption among children and adults today in America. Putting too much salt into your bloodstream causes the sodium-carbohydrate interaction and creates conditions for developing many other health problems.

(6)

EAT FOR GOOD HEALTH, AND TO FEEL GREAT

So far, you've learned about reconnecting with your authentic weight, how to recognize when you're eating for reasons other than being truly hungry, how to pay attention to your hunger and satiation signals, how to break out of old food habits by forming new neural pathways in your brain, and why grains and grain-flour foods are the most significant factor in unwanted weight gain. My focus in this chapter is on a variety of issues to remind you of the big picture behind your eating habits and your weight. In addition to rediscovering and achieving your authentic weight, *you want to eat to be in good health and to feel great.*

The better you feel about your weight every morning, the more optimistic, self-confident, and proud you will be. Your attitude toward life will improve, and you'll be happy to adhere to eating habits that help you achieve or maintain your authentic weight.

Let's take a look at more of the elements that contribute to embracing your authentic weight, eating for health, and feeling great.

Eat a Diverse Diet, Not a Balanced Diet

The most common advice you'll hear about eating healthy is "eat a balanced diet." What this usually means is that you should follow the U.S. Department of Agriculture (USDA) definition of eating from among five food groups: fruits, vegetables, grains, proteins, and dairy products. Many people still think of the government's advice in terms of the old "food pyramid." It suggested that, to have a balanced diet, you should eat a specific number of items from each category of the pyramid every day.

A major problem with this, however, is that people's nutritional needs change daily. My position is that the food pyramid is too generic. Plus, in the "balanced diet" concept, the nutrient amounts recommended are based on scientific studies of actual quantities people consumed over a period of time. The averages obtained through those kinds of studies are unreliable for a variety of reasons. The most significant of those is that, as an individual, your nutritional requirements depend completely on your own body's particular situation, which, again, varies on a day-to-day basis.

What is far better for your health is to eat a *diverse* diet, not a balanced diet. Did you know that the human body needs over one hundred different nutrients? There is no single food or food group that can provide all the necessary nutrients during one meal. Getting all those nutrients is why humans need to eat multiple meals composed of a wide variety of foods.

Fortunately, the USDA has recognized this. It replaced the concept of a pyramid with a different chart that gives almost equal weight to four of the five food groups, with the fifth group, dairy, smaller and literally outside of the chart. (Information on how to use this system can be found at MyPlate.gov.) This recommendation recognized that people should alter their eating habits daily to form a pattern of eating that supports optimum health. The government's *Dietary Guidelines for Americans (2020–2025)* holds that "everyone, no matter their age, race, or ethnicity, economic circumstances, or health status, can benefit from shifting food and beverage choices to better support healthy dietary patterns.... Researchers and public health experts understand that nutrients and foods are not consumed in isolation. Rather, people consume them in various combinations over time—a dietary pattern—and these foods and beverages act synergistically to affect health."

Eat a *diverse* diet, not a balanced diet. The human body needs over 100 different nutrients, and no single food or food group can provide all the necessary nutrients during one meal. This is why humans need to eat multiple meals composed of a wide variety of foods.

Instead of a "balanced diet," my emphasis is on variability. You want to eat a wide variety of foods to ensure that you're getting all the nutrients your body needs. Science has identified 118 nutrients that are used at some time for human health. Every food item you eat is a mixture of *macro-* and *micronutrients* existing in different combinations and ratios. Macronutrients are the larger, most common elements your body needs most. Micronutrients are those needed in small quantities but which are nevertheless important in cell metabolism. No one knows with certainty how much of each of these the body needs or how we derive them from the foods we eat. That is why I always suggest eating a diverse diet to improve your chances of consuming as many nutrients as possible.

Your best choice is to focus on eating a wide assortment of the freshest vegetables and fruits *in season in your region*, along with meat, fish, and dairy as you like. Eating according to the season helps ensure that the foods are the freshest with their nutrients intact, as opposed to canned and processed foods, which may have lowered levels of nutrients. Yes, you can also indulge in a small amount of carbohydrates such as bread, pasta, rice, and baked goods, but you must aim to minimize your consumption of these to less than 30% of your daily calories.

Some kids, most notably teenagers, refuse to eat vegetables and fruits, and some adults have a tendency to eat the same foods over and over. Do you have an overweight teen who has a limited eating scope? It may be difficult (if not impossible), but try to engage them in a discussion where you can point out that they're missing many nutrients their body needs. Add that a variety of foods will help them achieve and maintain a healthy weight. You can also model getting sufficient nutrients by varying your own diet.

Are you an adult who tends to eat the same things every week? Branch out and open your mind to checking out new fruits, vegetables, meats, and spices. Vary your menus by trying new recipes every week. Think of eating as a journey to explore the great diversity of nutrients available to humankind. Go online, where you can find thousands of easy-to-make recipes for busy adults, or buy a recipe magazine at the supermarket. Most bookstores have large cookbook collections and even your local library will have recipe books. I published *The Diabetes-Free Cookbook and Exercise Guide*, which contains over 80 recipes designed to help stabilize blood sugar; these recipes are delicious even if you are not diabetic.

Nearly all third-party weight loss programs fail in the long run. The moment participants stop using the prepackaged foods, they revert to their old unhealthy eating habits—and so they just regain the weight. Your internal regulatory system is a much better partner to beat weight gain than some external program of your food management.

You generally don't need to understand the nutrient composition of any food you're eating. Let your subconscious mind and conscious sensory controls guide you to what items to eat and how much to consume. If compelled to overeat to gain a particular micronutrient, your brain will help you terminate the meal when that need is met. It will then compensate for the excess intake of other nutrients during subsequent meals through cravings you may get for different foods.

The most significant requirements are that you eat in response to hunger and that you consume a variety of natural, unprocessed foods prepared simply to preserve their nutrient values.

DON'T RELY ON THIRD-PARTY WEIGHT LOSS PROGRAMS

Instead of learning to regulate and discipline yourself, you might be tempted to join one of the popular branded weight loss programs, often using prepackaged foods you purchase from them for all your meals. However, I strongly discourage you from doing that. You lose the opportunity to retrain your brain when you give the responsibility of determining what and how you eat to someone else. And retraining your brain is of the utmost importance, and the most effective way to make new habits stick.

Most importantly, understand that nearly all these third-party weight loss programs fail in the long run. The moment participants stop using the prepackaged foods, they go back to eating on their own where they revert to their old unhealthy eating habits—and so they just regain the weight.

Your internal regulatory system is a much better partner to beat weight gain than some external program of your food management. Doing this yourself, using the skills you're learning, will make you far more conscious of the right foods and how much of them to eat. Once you create new neural pathways in your brain, making new eating habits to beat unwanted weight gain becomes easier and more enjoyable.

Learn to Read Food Labels

Unless you never buy any type of packaged or canned food, you're going to encounter the government-required label on food items. The information provided has changed over time to the point that many adults don't actually understand it. The result is that a lot of people are buying unhealthy foods that are counterproductive to losing weight.

Let's take a look at how to read a food label, using one for packaged bread and one for pasta sauce as examples:

BREAD

Nutrition Facts

8 servings per container

Serving size	**1/8 Bread (57g)**
Amount per serving	
Calories	**170**
	% Daily Value*
Total Fat 2g	3%
Saturated Fat 1g	5%
Trans Fat 0g	
Cholesterol 0mg	0%
Sodium 300mg	13%
Total Carbohydrate 31g	11%
Dietary Fiber 2g	7%
Total Sugars 3g	
Includes 2g Added Sugars	4%
Protein 6g	
Vitamin D 1mcg	6%
Calcium10mg	0%
Iron 2mg	10%
Potassium 70mg	2%

*The % Daily Value tells you how much a nutrient in a serving of food contributes to a daily diet. 2,000 calories a day is used for general nutrition advice.

PASTA SAUCE

Nutrition Facts

5 servings per container

Serving size	**1/2 Cup (125g)**
Amount per serving	
Calories	**100**
	% Daily Value*
Total Fat 7g	9%
Saturated Fat 1g	5%
Trans Fat 0g	
Cholesterol 0mg	0%
Sodium 420mg	18%
Total Carbohydrate 6g	2%
Dietary Fiber 1g	5%
Total Sugars 4g	
Includes0g Added Sugars	0%
Protein 2g	
Vitamin D 0 mcg	0%
Calcium 20mg	0%
Iron 0.2mg	0%
Potassium 307mg	8%

*The % Daily Value tells you how much a nutrient in a serving of food contributes to a daily diet. 2,000 calories a day is used for general nutrition advice.

Servings per container and serving size: Each product label states how many servings the package contains and the serving size. You must always check this first, as the rest of the information on the label is per serving. Some small packages of products can fool you into thinking they're low in carbohydrates and sodium, until you notice the many servings they supposedly contain. If you consume most or all the contents of a can or package, you must multiply the percentages by the number of servings you ate.

Calories: The number of calories per serving is displayed. If you're aiming to lose weight, it can be useful to lower your total daily intake of calories. However, most people are simply unable to track their calorie intake throughout the entire day, and I'm not a proponent of calorie counting. Instead, this book has encouraged you to pay attention to your brain telling you what foods to eat as well as learning to monitor your own portion size. It's extremely difficult for most adults to count calories for months on end, so learning how much food to eat is your best method of avoiding weight gain.

% Daily Value: The U.S. Food and Drug Administration has already determined how much of each nutrient on the food label you should consume each day. The food label thus tells you the percentage of that nutrient that is provided in a single serving. But the problem with trying to track your total daily consumption of every nutrient is similar to counting calories—it's just very difficult to track all these items every day for months and months if you're trying to beat weight gain. Even if you try to keep a diary of your food intake, it takes a lot of time and you are likely to miss recording some meals. My recommendation is, again, listen to your brain, pay attention to your hunger and satiation signals, relearn what portion size is adequate for you, and eat a diverse diet. (Note: Be aware also of the fact that "% daily values" listed on food labels do not take into account children. If you are trying to help your child avoid weight gain, that information is not very useful to you.)

Total Fat: This information reveals how much fat is in the product, broken down into saturated fat (which can clog arteries) and trans fat. The American Heart Association recommends no more than 13 grams of saturated fat per day. Trans fat is created by adding hydrogen to vegetable oils to make them more solid. Companies use trans fats to make processed foods last longer. Avoid products with trans fats.

Cholesterol: Dietary cholesterol comes from animal products you consume, including eggs, high-fat and processed meats, dairy products, and baked goods made with eggs, butter, and cream. Prior guidelines recommended consuming very little dietary cholesterol to avoid heart disease. However, food scientists have expanded their view of the former limits and now simply recommend keeping your consumption of products with dietary cholesterol low.

The next time you go grocery shopping, check the labels of the items that you may have been using for years. Are any of them extremely high in carbohydrates, sodium, or added sugars? If yes, they may have contributed to your weight gain and perhaps it's time to stop purchasing them.

Sodium: Reading labels to check the sodium content is a must. As discussed in Chapter 5, high levels of sodium in your diet add to your cravings for carbs. Aim to keep your sodium consumption between 1200 and 1500 milligrams per day. Some breads, many canned vegetables, pickles, and jarred pasta sauces often contain a huge amount of sodium per serving, as do snack foods.

Carbohydrates: As we discussed in Chapter 5, avoiding or at least reducing your consumption of foods high in carbohydrates is a non-debatable key to losing weight. A single slice of bread often contains between 18 and 40 grams of carbohydrate. Since each 4 grams of carbohydrate equals 1 teaspoon of sugar, a slice of bread can have the effect of about 4 to 10 teaspoons of sugar. A sandwich with two slices of bread doubles that. So be sure to read the labels on the breads and many types of processed foods you buy to see how much carbohydrate is in them.

Note also that labels display three sub-categories under carbohydrates:

> *Fiber:* Grains and vegetables that contain carbohydrates also provide fiber. This information shows you how much fiber is included in the carbohydrate total.
>
> *Total Sugars:* Some carbs in foods are sugars, so this number shows you how many grams of sugar are part of the carbohydrate count.
>
> *Includes Added Sugars:* Some products contain sugars, such as honey, maple syrup, and other sweeteners. Companies add these to sweeten a food item or to extend its shelf life. Avoid foods with added sugars.

Protein: This information displays the protein content of the food item. Note that many foods provide protein, not just meats. Legumes such as lentils and many types of beans are rich in protein, so add them to your diet rather than eating meat with every meal. Vegetarians usually include legumes in their diet to meet much of their protein needs.

Vitamin and mineral content: Below the solid line on food labels are listed the vitamins and minerals contained in a single serving of the food.

×××

The next time you go grocery shopping, check the labels of the items that you may have been using for years. Are any of them extremely high in carbohydrates, sodium, or added sugars? If yes, they may have contributed to your weight gain over the years, and perhaps it's time to stop purchasing them. To change the old neural pathways guiding your food-shopping habits, begin looking for new foods with more nutritious value that you can substitute. Transform your grocery shopping into an activity that makes you feel healthy and fit as you beat unwanted weight gain.

Two Habits to Shed: No-Calorie (Sugar-Free) Sweeteners and Smoothies

The following advice may surprise you, but here it is. If you're serious about feeling good about yourself and losing weight, I propose that you avoid two habits that are part of the lifestyle of many people.

The first is using no-calorie sugar-free sweeteners made from alternative plants or artificial chemicals. No-calorie sweeteners for your coffee, iced tea, or baking can seem like the perfect solution to avoid adding sugar. But, as we discussed in Chapter 5, natural sugar is not the major culprit in weight gain. To avoid gaining weight, your main emphasis needs to be on reducing your consumption of grains and grain-flour products.

There are three problems with no-calorie sweeteners. First, you may falsely assume you're helping yourself lose weight. But the calorie "savings" of no-calorie sweeteners could cause you to eat more of other foods, especially high-carb items. Have you ever noticed someone who used a no-calorie sugar substitute in their coffee but then ate a large Danish or muffin? Are you one of those people?

BEWARE OF "ADDED SUGARS" IN DRINKS

In recent years. there has been a tidal wave of beverages produced with added sugar, often high-fructose corn syrup. Such taste-enhancing additives are a major contributing factor to the increasing cases of obesity in the U.S. and throughout the world. The proof of this is the astonishing statistic that Americans consume an average of 22 teaspoons of added sugar per day! And most of it is in the form of soda and sweetened drinks.

You may not realize the enormous amount of sugar in these drinks. While an 8-ounce glass of milk contains about 3 teaspoons of sugar (in the form of lactose), there are 8 teaspoons of sugar in a can of regular soda. If the beverage you drink is sweetened at a concentration above what's natural, the brain has no mechanism to regulate how much you need to drink to satisfy your thirst. I recommend weaning yourself off sodas and beverages with added sugar or high fructose corn syrup to reduce your sugar intake.

Second, no-calorie sweeteners skew your taste buds' sense of sweetness, which confuses your brain. When it gets the signal of a sweet taste in the mouth, the brain expects that glucose will soon be delivered. But artificial sweeteners deliver no energy that the body can use. After consuming a no-calorie sweetener, the brain's inability to predict what should happen to your blood glucose level could cause it to start misinterpreting the results of eating real sugars in the future.

Third, the prolonged use of no-calorie sweeteners can cause you to lose the sensation of sweetness when you eat naturally sweet edibles—such as fruit. You then enter a not-sweet-enough zone for a lot of foods. Essentially, you have become accustomed to the intensity of a no-calorie sweetener, and the taste of natural sugar is no longer enough. To compensate, you might even start adding no-calorie sweeteners to more foods, perpetuating the problem.

In short, I say stay away from no-calorie sweeteners. They're not compatible with your goal of working with your brain's natural capabilities to help you reach and maintain your authentic weight.

The second habit to avoid is making, buying, and drinking smoothies—a trend that has become a fad among many U.S. teens and adults. When you drink blended or pureed foods, you have little control over how much you consume before you feel satisfied. You tend to drink an entire glass or more of the smoothie before your brain can ascertain the nutrient content of each mouthful. This is in contrast to when you chew the foods. You may think it's a good idea to get a lot of different nutrients by blending an assortment of fruits and/or vegetables; but it's actually an easy way to end up overconsuming carbohydrates. If you want to lose weight, cut back on how often you drink smoothies.

When you drink blended or pureed foods, you have little control over how much you consume before you feel satisfied. You tend to drink an entire glass or more of the smoothie before your brain can ascertain the nutrient content of each mouthful. You may think it's a good idea to get a lot of different nutrients by blending an assortment of fruits and/or vegetables; but it's actually an easy way to end up overconsuming carbohydrates. If you want to lose weight, cut back on how often you drink smoothies.

Moderate Your Consumption of Alcohol

Many adults in America enjoy alcohol in the form of beer, wine, and spirits. Before dinner, drinks stimulate your appetite and enliven social events. Wine and beer often complement the taste of food. Alcohol tends to make people feel happier and less stressed.

But, on the downside, some types of alcohol—or just drinking too much alcohol—can play a role in weight gain. Here's a little chemistry about alcohol that explains why.

Typically, beer is 3 to 8% ethanol (alcohol) by volume. Wines have 10 to 15%, and spirits have up to 40% alcohol by volume. The molecules of alcohol you consume are changed in the liver. The resulting chemicals can be utilized in the same metabolic way that cells use glucose for their energy production. And the body tends to use these chemicals first. This means that millions of glucose molecules that would have been used for cellular energy production can remain unused. They stay in the liver or float in the bloodstream. In addition, beers and wines also contribute sugars that add to glucose levels. Much of this excess glucose is converted to fat to be stored in your fat cells. A lot of this glucose goes to fat cells in readily available areas—think "beer belly"—as well as being a factor in high blood sugar.

When people drink alcohol, especially in a social setting, they also tend to munch on snacks like salty chips, crackers, and cheese, or hors d'oeuvres that contain carbohydrates. This means that consuming alcohol can be a double whammy to your carb consumption, leading to weight gain.

If you sometimes join friends for happy hour, or love to sip a great wine with dinner or relax with a few beers watching a ballgame, you don't need to severely restrict your enjoyment of alcohol. But you do need to be totally honest with yourself. Are you gaining weight or failing to shed pounds even though you've made adjustments in your diet? If so, you might consider whether your alcohol consumption is a contributing factor.

As long as you're trying to make changes in the amount and type of food you consume, why not consider altering your alcohol intake in your new lifestyle? You may see a difference in both your weight and how you feel about yourself when you take a new approach to drinking alcohol. And consider these guidelines from the U.S. government for moderate alcohol consumption. They recommend no more than two servings of alcohol a day or less for men, and one serving or less daily for women. They also make the point that drinking less is better for your overall health.

One way to drink less without sacrificing enjoyment is to sip your drink rather than gulping it. The enjoyment of drinking actually comes from a thin layer of molecules that coats the taste buds on your tongue. When you drink in gulps, most of the liquid goes straight down your throat after flowing over your taste bud sensors. By sipping, you will still get the full enjoyment of the beer, wine, or alcohol while reducing the quantity that goes into your body.

Feed Your Gut Bacteria to Lose Weight

Yes, this section on losing weight and feeling healthy is indeed about feeding the bacteria in your colon (large intestine). What do bacteria have to do with these things? Quite a lot, as you'll see. Let me start by talking about the role of gut bacteria in maintaining good health.

First, your colon contains about four hundred types of bacteria, both beneficial and harmful ones. Bacteria began growing right from your infancy, introduced during breast feeding or other milk or food you consumed.

What does good bacteria have to do with weight gain? Your intestinal bacteria need many nutrients for themselves and also produce many nutrients the body needs. If the beneficial bacteria in the intestine are not fed and protected, the brain may create cravings for foods that in your past contained that particular nutrient. You can end up eating extra food that results in weight gain.

By the age of two and a half, your intestinal bacteria already resemble that of an adult in terms of composition, and this usually remains stable until old age. This wide variety of intestinal bacteria comes from the many types of food you eat.

Your gut needs a prevalence of good bacteria to crowd out the bad bacteria and to ensure they don't get enough nutrients to take over. Good gut bacteria perform many functions. They produce nutrients needed for the maintenance of the intestinal wall lining. Without a healthy intestinal wall, you couldn't absorb needed nutrients into your bloodstream. Furthermore, a strong intestinal wall prevents incompletely digested proteins from getting into the body, which would create the potential for an autoimmune response.

Healthy bacteria in the gut are also essential for normal brain function. The gut produces approximately 90% of the *serotonin* that helps nerve cells communicate with each other. In addition, two neurochemicals, *noradrenaline* and *dopamine,* are generated by nerve cells using precursor molecules made by gut bacteria. Thus, gut bacteria influence brain mechanisms that regulate normal brain activities, including memory and the release of stress hormones. A 2019 review of studies of gut bacteria in patients with depression showed that at least fifty types of gut bacterial species differed from those of control subjects without depression.

Finally, good gut bacteria are essential for the performance of two components of your immune system:

4 WAYS TO SUPPORT GOOD GUT BACTERIA

Here are some ways you can improve your diet to ensure you have an abundance of good bacteria.

- ***Consume prebiotics.*** These compounds are nondigestible in the small intestine, so they feed the colon (large intestine) bacteria. You can find various products now that contain prebiotics.
- ***Consume probiotics.*** Another solution to boost healthy gut bacteria is to consume foods that contain probiotics. These are live microorganisms that confer health benefits to you by improving your intestinal microbial balance. Fermented products that contain lactic acid bacteria—such as yogurt, kefir, and buttermilk—are prime examples. Various drinks, such as kombucha, are made with as many as billions of probiotics, as well. Some studies suggest that probiotics have a beneficial effect, especially for people with depression and anxiety.
- ***Eat fresh vegetables and foods that contain "resistant starches."*** Resistant starch occurs naturally in chicory, garlic, leeks, seeds, and legumes, such as beans and lentils.

prevention and protection. In terms of prevention, a molecule called *lactoferrin* in milk, saliva, tears, and nasal secretions has antimicrobial capabilities and prevents the attachment of *H. pylori* (*Helicobacter pylori*) to the stomach wall. *H. pylori* is a bacteria that can cause ulcers, gastritis, and stomach cancer. Meanwhile, the body achieves immune protection by producing antibodies and white blood cells, also called immune cells. During an infection, millions of new immune cells are created to replace old ones. Such newly minted immune cells need to learn how to recognize normal cells in the body so they don't attack them.

Resistant starch may also be added as part of dried raw foods or used as an additive in manufactured foods. The benefit of resistant starch is that it's not digested in the small intestine, so it provides nourishment for the good bacteria in the large intestine, and this helps them thrive. Some people find it uncomfortable to eat the foods cited above, as they contain *inulins* that are indigestible by the enzymes that normally digest starch. As a result, gut bacteria metabolize them, releasing carbon dioxide, hydrogen, and methane, causing bloating and flatulence. You can mediate the effects of these foods by taking medications containing simethicone, which promotes the coalescence of smaller bubbles into larger ones that are more easily passed from the body.

- ***Limit your consumption of the grains and grain-flour products.*** This includes wheat, corn, and rice. These complex carbohydrates often require salt to improve their taste, and this creates the environment in which *H. pylori* thrives. As cited above, this can damage the lining of the stomach and lead to infection and the further production of bad bacteria.

Bacteria in the gut, carrying markers similar to normal cells in the body, train those immune cells to identify infectious agents in the body. This type of training prevents autoimmune diseases. Therefore, nourishing the normal bacterial colony in your gut is an important function that helps you maintain a robust immune system.

So, what does good bacteria have to do with weight gain? Your intestinal bacteria need many nutrients for themselves and also produce many nutrients the body needs. If the beneficial bacteria in the intestine are not fed and protected, the brain may create cravings for foods that in your past contained that particular nutrient. You can end up eating extra food that results in weight gain.

Mindful Lifestyle, Mindful Eating

My last recommendation about eating for health and feeling great is to take a mindfulness approach to both eating and life in general. Mindfulness is a "mindset" with roots in age-old Eastern philosophies. The practice involves creating a deep awareness of a present situation. In recent years, it's been applied to pain management, anxiety, and substance abuse, but I suggest it can also be applied to weight management.

At its core, mindful eating is about being fully conscious of and reconnecting with how you're choosing to eat. Take, for example, the *speed* at which you eat. Eating slowly and consciously is, in my view, one of the ultimate keys to health and controlling your weight. Mindfulness helps you stay connected to your authentic weight by paying attention to your hunger and satiation signals and being more conscious of your chewing.

In our fast-paced lives, most people tend to eat very quickly. Working people often gulp down their breakfast and lunch in an attempt to save time. Even family dinners can be rushed because everyone has to get to some evening activity. So many people just gobble down their food without being truly aware of their eating habits. They're not truly appreciating the food; nor are they really enjoying it.

At its core, mindful eating is about being fully conscious of and reconnecting with how you're choosing to eat. Take, for example, the *speed* at which you eat. Eating slowly and consciously is, in my view, one of the ultimate keys to health and controlling your weight. Mindfulness helps you stay connected to your authentic weight by paying attention to your hunger and satiation signals and being more conscious of your chewing.

Eating fast is not a natural way to consume food, and it tends to encourage you to overeat by taking second helpings when you don't need them.

Is this you? Do you dash through your meals? Perhaps you speed-eat over the kitchen table or even the kitchen counter at home at times? Do you cram the food down quickly at your desk during lunch at work?

One consequence of hurrying through meals is that it doesn't allow time to chew your food sufficiently. As discussed earlier, chewing slowly is important for conveying data to the brain regarding the nutrients you're taking in. You also need to slow down in order to stay in touch with your hunger and "stop eating" signals. Rushed meals are hard on your digestion, too.

Your goal should be to taste every bite of food as it passes through your mouth. Here's how to slow down:

- First, experience the qualities of the food in your mouth by taking smaller bites and taking time to chew them.
- Second, decide whether or not the food is appealing before, during, and after chewing.
- Third, swallow the food.
- If the food begins to no longer be appealing, take that as a sign that you have likely eaten enough.

Each time you eat too fast to really enjoy the food, you continue to reinforce that old neural pathway and this unwanted behavior. Take time now to slow down and truly appreciate the variety of flavors and textures that you take into your mouth during meals. As you mindfully choose to eat slowly, you'll develop this as a new healthy habit that has many benefits.

Mindfully Focus on Your Meals

The practice of mindful eating is also about focusing your attention only on your meal. Listening to the radio or reading a magazine while eating makes it difficult for the brain to regulate your intake based on sensory signals. The importance of this cannot be underestimated. Try to eat your meals in a calm, peaceful environment without distractions so you can consciously focus on what you eat, how it tastes, and how much you're consuming.

Although the brain is capable of multitasking, this doesn't produce optimal performance. Magnetic resonance imaging studies show that total brain activity decreases when people try to concentrate simultaneously on two demanding tasks. In short, distracted eating can easily lead to weight gain because the brain isn't in touch with the amount of food you're taking in.

When you pay attention to TV news during a meal, for instance, your awareness of eating is handed off to the subconscious part of your brain. Although your subconscious may also process the signals coming from the taste and smell receptors, your conscious mind is focused on the TV, not on the loss of enjoyment or the incoming signals of satiation. Because of this, your conscious mind cannot control how much you consume and you'll tend to overeat.

If you want to be confident in your ability to control your portions and the amount of food you consume—no matter how pleasing it looks or how good it smells—practice mindful eating. Aim to not be distracted during meals. You'll be better able to engage your brain's full attention during mealtimes in order to beat unwanted weight gain.

Finally, I suggest that you apply mindfulness to many elements in your life. If you're gaining weight or unable to lose it, it may mean that you're just not paying enough attention to your lifestyle as a whole. Perhaps you're stressed or depressed and use food to calm yourself. Perhaps you're rushing through life, not appreciating the beauty around you or your friends and family. The more you practice mindful eating, the more you might find your life improves in many other areas as well.

Key Points

- Instead of aiming for a *balanced* diet, put your emphasis on eating a *diverse* diet, with lots of variability. That's the real key. You want to eat a wide variety of foods to ensure that you're getting all the nutrients your body needs. The human body needs over one hundred different nutrients, and there is no single food or food group that can provide all the necessary nutrients during one meal.

- You might be tempted to sign up for one of the popular corporate weight loss programs—along with their prepackaged foods. However, I strongly discourage you from doing that. You lose the opportunity to retrain your brain when you give the responsibility of determining what and how you eat to someone else.
- Learn how to read food labels. Then when you go grocery shopping, check the labels of the items that you may have been using for years. Are any of them extremely high in carbohydrates, sodium, or added sugars? If so, begin looking for new foods with more nutritious value that you can substitute.
- I recommend weaning yourself off sodas and beverages with added sugar or high fructose corn syrup to reduce your sugar intake. You may not realize the enormous amount of sugar in these drinks.
- If you're serious about feeling good about yourself and losing weight, I propose that you avoid two habits that are part of the lifestyle of many people. The first is using no-calorie sugar-free sweeteners made from alternative plants or artificial chemicals. The second habit is making or buying smoothies—a trend that has become a fad among many U.S. teens and adults.

- As long as you're trying to make changes in the amount and type of food you consume, why not include altering your alcohol intake in your new lifestyle? You may see a difference in your weight and how you feel about yourself when you take a new approach to drinking alcohol. Drinking every day or drinking a lot of alcohol each time you imbibe may have a real effect on your inability to get control of your weight.
- To lose weight and feel healthy, you'll want to understand how to support the bacteria in your colon (large intestine). Bacteria in the gut have a lot to do with both.
- As an important part of a mindful eating approach, eating slowly and consciously is perhaps one of the ultimate keys to health. The practice of mindful eating is also about focusing your attention only on your meal. Finally, I suggest that you apply mindfulness to other elements of your life. In addition to speeding through meals, you may also be rushing through life.

(7)

EXERCISE TO STAY HEALTHY, NOT TO LOSE WEIGHT

In almost every book on weight management, exercise is usually mentioned as the key to losing weight and keeping it off. On the surface, you would think this makes good biological sense. Here's what is commonly believed to happen when you exercise. First, your muscles send a message to the brain for additional fuel. The brain, in turn, sends a signal to the liver to release glucose to supply fuel to muscles. In addition, the brain sends another message to your fat cells to release more fatty acids that can be burned as fuel. Given this biology, it's thought that we are emptying our fat cells—and losing weight.

However, this scenario is not exactly accurate. It's true that many people, especially those young in age, can lose weight using exercise as a tool. But this is not true for everyone at every age.

Frankly, I have a completely different view of exercise that I believe is important enough to bring to your attention. This chapter is actually about a paradox you need to understand. This seventh way to beat weight gain is actually a sort of warning that you *cannot* count on exercise as a method to shed pounds. The crux of my advice here is:

As losing weight from exercise alone is unlikely, focus on exercising for optimum health.

Let's look at why I say this and what you can do to ensure you maximize the benefits you get from exercising.

Why You Shouldn't Count on Exercise for Weight Loss

First, most people simply don't exercise enough to accomplish the goal of emptying their fat cells. Exercising burns very few calories relative to one's daily food intake, especially if you're already overeating. Consider these statistics about how many calories a woman weighing 140 pounds will burn in these various activities:

- Walking: 270 calories by walking 3.5 miles in one hour
- Biking: 90 calories by riding a bike for 10 to 12 miles in one hour
- Running: 430 calories by running 30 minutes at a speed of 7.5 mph

Now apply those calorie burns to a diet of 1800 or 2000 calories per day. You can see that this woman will barely make a dent in depleting her fat cells and losing weight. This is true even if she exercises seven days per week. Although the numbers are just slightly different for a man weighing 160 or 180 pounds, the small impact of exercising on losing weight is the exactly same.

Add the fact that exercise itself usually makes people feel hungrier. You go out for a walk, a bike ride, or to the gym, after which you return home and eat more than usual. You tell yourself you've "worked up an appetite." Exercise often makes people crave sweets or think they deserve a reward of ice cream or cookies. If your strenuous exercise regimen is accompanied by *increased* calorie intake, you might end up gaining weight rather than losing it.

Exercise is usually thought of as a key to losing weight and keeping it off. On the surface, you would think this makes good biological sense. But you cannot count on exercise as a method to shed pounds, especially for people over 50 when it's very difficult to keep up the level of activity needed to lose weight with aging muscles.

One of the most unrecognized problems is that exercise has a decreasing effect on weight loss as you age. For most people over 50, it's very difficult to keep up the level of activity needed to lose weight with aging muscles. What used to take 20 minutes to burn 300 calories now takes 40 minutes or even an hour. This is because people begin losing muscle and muscle function as they age. Less muscle, less burning of calories.

Let me sum it up this way. If exercise were truly necessary for weight control, everyone who's eating but not exercising should keep on gaining weight, but not everyone does. For example, we don't see every senior citizen who eats continue gaining weight, given that seniors typically slow down in their activities. And if exercise were the body's natural mechanism to maintain weight, then we would all feel the urge to exercise after a sumptuous meal—just as we feel the urge to move when listening to music with a strong beat. Instead, most of us feel lethargic after a heavy meal.

SPECIAL NOTE FOR MEN ABOUT EXERCISING AS YOU AGE

Men, please take note of this fact. You will lose muscle mass in the legs and arms as you go into your 60s, 70s, and 80s. This means you have less muscle burning calories. This is a reflection of the increasing divergence between your ability to extract energy from food versus the energy you use during your daily activities. Although your efficiency in extracting energy from food doesn't change significantly throughout your lifetime, your efficiency in using this energy to do muscle work is increasingly reduced due to the effects of reduced hormones in the body, which results in reduced muscle mass. This is fairly well publicized for women in menopause, but the same thing is true for men also. Yes, there is male menopause that results in a lower level of hormones.

What Exercise Is Good For

If exercising isn't an effective method to lose weight, why did I include it in this book? The answer is, I want to encourage you to exercise because exercise keeps your body healthy in many other ways. It stimulates your brain and keeps you feeling fit, energetic, and youthful. In my view, these are all ingredients of the self-awareness you want to have in order to get and stay connected to your authentic weight. In short, exercise improves your attitude about yourself and inspires you to follow the other six recommendations in this book.

Here's how exercise helps you at any age. First, the primary objective of exercise is to condition the lungs, heart, and muscles, regardless of your body weight. Such conditioning develops reserve capacity available for use when you need it and when you become sick. For example, an older person who doesn't exercise may have the capacity to deliver from the lungs one liter of oxygen per minute to the tissues, plus a reserve capacity of three to four liters per minute. In contrast, a more fit older person who does exercise may have twice that much reserve. Furthermore, when a fit older person develops a condition, such as pneumonia, he or she has more available respiratory reserves. The same is true of a conditioned heart in a fit older individual—it can pump more blood with less effort than one in an unconditioned person. Exercising can thus help you through a serious illness.

I encourage you to exercise because exercise keeps your body healthy in many ways. It stimulates your brain and keeps you feeling fit, energetic, and youthful. These are all ingredients of the self-awareness you want to have in order to get and stay connected to your authentic weight. Exercise improves your attitude about yourself and inspires you to follow the recommendations in this book.

Exercising also helps your muscles and other organs. For instance, conditioning allows your muscles to work longer before your brain senses the stress of exercising and makes you feel tired. Additional benefits of exercise come from improved blood circulation, which helps the brain think more creatively and the skin to have a better tone. The sustained elevation of body temperature you get from exercise also improves your immune system and the defense mechanisms of the body. Exercising also helps keep your core and back muscles in shape, which helps prevent falls as you age.

For many people, the addition of exercise in their daily routines also reduces stress and offers the key to greater psychological happiness and well-being, even if they're gaining weight or only losing it slowly.

Finally, if you're diagnosed with prediabetes or diabetes, exercise can help your muscles burn more fatty acids as well as glucose, thereby reducing their levels in your blood. It has been shown that regular exercise promotes the storage of more fat in fat cells under the skin, keeping it away from the blood stream.

What Type of Exercise Should You Do?

What type or types of exercise you should do is largely up to each person—based on your age, past experience with exercising, your geographic location, your weather, and other factors. In general, you want to do aerobic exercise, which increases your heart rate and blood flow.

Walking is one of the best and easiest forms of aerobic exercise that anyone can do, no matter your age or where you live. You don't need to walk the proverbial 8000 steps per day; about 5000 steps is sufficient. This is about two miles, and it can be done in roughly 30 to 40 minutes of walking. You can walk outside, in a mall, or on a treadmill.

Doing some weight training is worthwhile to keep your muscles conditioned. You can go to a gym or buy various weights to work with at home. Well-conditioned muscles also help in burning more calories.

There is, of course, a wide range of other activities you can do for exercise, including jogging, swimming, tennis, basketball, or the newest trend, pickleball.

Many people enroll in yoga classes, which is fine. Yoga is very beneficial for stretching and maintaining flexibility and balance as you age, as well as for stress reduction. But yoga is an anaerobic form of exercise, meaning it does not, in general, increase heart rate as do walking, running, biking, and so on.

So, although exercise alone is not the key to losing weight, please do incorporate an exercise habit into your lifestyle of living as healthfully as possible. If you are not accustomed to exercising, be sure to check with your doctor to make sure the exercise you plan to do is safe and appropriate, or if you have any concerns about exercising or a medical condition that might preclude certain types of exercise.

Key Points

- It's possible to lose weight through exercise, but most people can't rely on exercise as their primary method to lose or maintain weight.
- Exercising burns very few calories relative to one's daily food intake, especially if you're already overeating.
- Exercise is extremely valuable for one's health. Among the many benefits of exercise, it conditions the lungs, heart, and muscles, and improves blood circulation.
- Exercise can improve your confidence and awareness of your body, inspiring you to lose weight by following the other six recommendations in this book.

CONCLUSION

I hope you have enjoyed reading this book and have already started to implement my recommendations in your daily life. I truly want every reader of *Beat Unwanted Weight Gain* to live a healthier life at their authentic weight. There is no escape from the fact that unhealthy weight and obesity are on the rise in the U.S. (and in many countries around the world)—and the consequences on people's health and lifespan are serious.

Whatever your age, the seven recommendations I have made will help you in your commitment to achieving your weight loss goals. When you rediscover and maintain your authentic weight, you'll find yourself having more energy, feeling better about yourself, and finally enjoying one of the most meaningful activities of life—eating to feel healthy. Each meal will become an experience that allows you to feel in control of your life.

If there's one change I hope you'll make immediately, it's to become far more conscious of your eating habits—when you eat, whether you're hungry, what foods you're choosing, the portion sizes you're serving yourself, how much you're eating, and when you decide to stop eating.

As you practice all these elements of mindful eating, you'll find yourself automatically eating better and enjoying it more. Every time you're tempted to eat, you'll remember to ask yourself if you're truly hungry—or whether you're eating out of stress or for another reason. When you eat, you'll remember to chew your food thoroughly and become more aware of the flavors, spices, textures, and other unique qualities. You'll pay attention to when each bite no longer tastes as good as the first, telling you it's time to stop eating.

> **If there's one change I hope you'll make immediately, it's to become far more conscious of your eating habits. You can retrain your brain and take charge of your health. You can become conscious of your eating behavior. You can develop the willpower to resist the powerful marketing of unhealthy food in our culture and cultivate a lifestyle in which you're in control of your weight and your health.**

You can retrain your brain and become conscious of your eating behavior. You can develop the willpower to resist the powerful marketing of unhealthy food in our culture and cultivate a lifestyle in which you're in control.

Being in touch with your body and controlling your weight are two of the most important keys to healthy aging. The more aware you are of your nutritional needs, the better you'll be at self-regulating your eating behaviors. As your energy needs change over time, you'll be better at sensing how much you need to eat to avoid excessive weight gain. Using the recommendations in the seven chapters in this book, you'll grow older, but you will not grow fat or obese. You may slow down, but you'll feel healthy and capable.

Here's to your successful journey to your authentic weight and better health!

Sincerely,
Dr. John

Postscript: The more you understand how to maintain your own health, the better the chances that you will live a healthier, disease-free, long and happy life. Helping people is why I have committed decades to researching, writing, and publishing books on preventing weight gain and obesity, reversing Type 2 diabetes, surviving cancer, and recognizing medical disinformation. I invite you to take a deeper dive into learning more about these topics in my other books, as profiled on the following pages.

Finally, please visit my website, DrJohnOnHealth.com, to follow my blogs and to send me your questions or feedback on how this book has changed your life.

If you enjoyed this book or received value from it, would you be kind enough to leave a review of it on Amazon or Goodreads? It would be greatly appreciated!

ABOUT THE AUTHOR

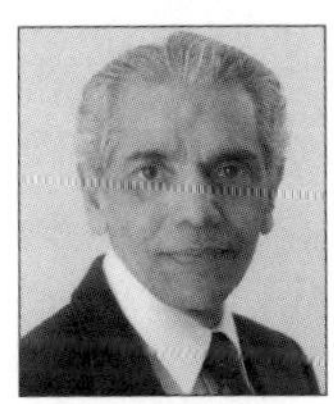

JOHN M. POOTHULLIL, MD, FCRP practiced medicine as a pediatrician and allergist for more than thirty years, most of those years in the state of Texas. He received his medical degree from the University of Kerala, India in 1968, after which he did two years of medical residency in Washington, D.C. and Phoenix, Arizona, and two years of fellowship, one in Milwaukee, Wisconsin and the other in Ontario, Canada. He began his practice in 1974 and retired in 2008. He holds certifications from the American Board of Pediatrics, The American Board of Allergy and Immunology, and the Canadian Board of Pediatrics.

During his medical practice, Dr. Poothullil became interested in understanding the causes of and interconnections between hunger, satiation, and weight gain. His interest turned into a passion and a multi-decade personal study and research project that led him to read widely many scholarly works in biology, biochemistry, physiology, endocrinology, and cellular metabolic functions. This eventually guided him to investigate the theory of insulin resistance as it relates to diabetes. Recognizing that this theory was illogical, he spent several years rethinking the biology behind high blood sugar and developed the fatty acid burn theory as the real cause of diabetes.

Dr. Poothullil has written articles on hunger and satiation, weight loss, diabetes, and the senses of taste and smell. His articles have been published in many peer-reviewed medical journals, including *Physiology & Behavior, Neuroscience & Biobehavioral Reviews, Journal of Women's Health, The Journal of Applied Research, Nutrition,* and *Nutritional Neuroscience.* His work has been quoted in *Woman's Day, Fitness, Redbook,* and *Woman's World.*

Dr. Poothullil is the author of seven books, including this one.

Please visit the website DrJohnOnHealth.com to follow Dr. Poothullil's blog and to send us your questions and feedback on how this book has changed your life.

OTHER BOOKS BY DR. POOTHULLIL

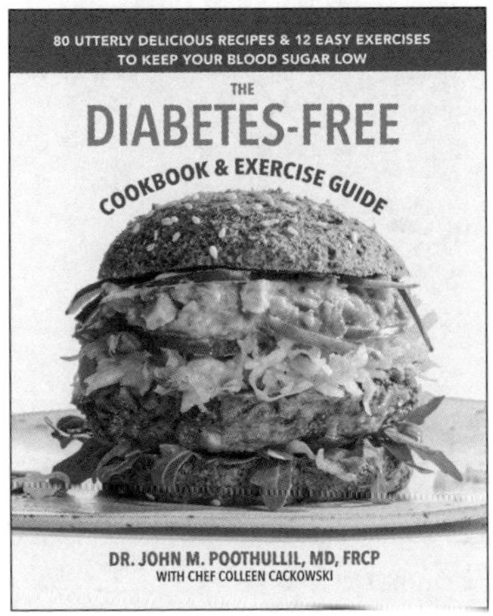

The Diabetes-Free Cookbook and Exercise Guide

Discover how you can live a diabetes-free life with Dr. John's groundbreaking cookbook and exercise guide. With over 80 appetizing low-carb recipes created by Chef Colleen Cackowski, you'll never miss the high-carb, high-sugar foods of your past. Every recipe nourishes your body and keeps your blood sugar levels in check so you can enjoy tasty, satisfying meals. Dr. John also offers 12 easy-to-do exercises to boost your flexibility and balance and keep you healthy as you age.

Winner: Small Press Books, Eric Hoffer Book Awards
Finalist: Cookbooks, Next Generation Indie Book Awards

New Insights Press

ISBN: 979-8-9860163-4-4 (Hardcover)
ISBN: 979-8-9860163-7-5 (eBook)

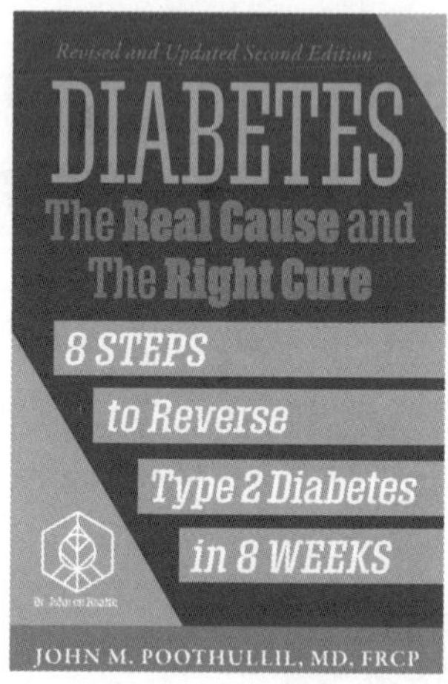

Diabetes: The Real Cause and the Right Cure, 2nd Edition: 8 Steps to Reverse Type 2 Diabetes in 8 Weeks

NEW EDITION—Whether you were recently diagnosed or have had Type 2 diabetes for years, this book will open your eyes to new thinking about the real cause and an actual cure based on scientific thinking. If you think that diabetes is your destiny because it is in your family, this book will show you that this thinking is not true. The fact is, you can reverse high blood sugar and diabetes in as little as 8 weeks using the 8 steps in this book.

New Insights Press

ISBN: 979-8986016382 (Paperback)
ISBN: 979-8986016399 (eBook)

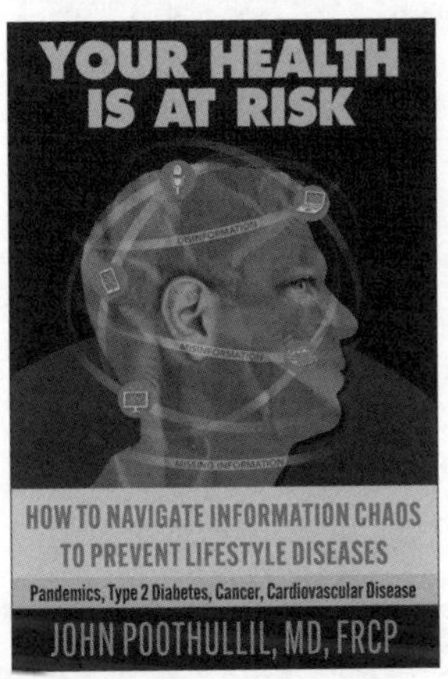

Your Health Is at Risk: How to Navigate Information Chaos to Prevent Lifestyle Diseases

This book explains how medical disinformation, misinformation, and missing Information (DMMI) are increasingly pervasive in the media and social media, leading you to make poor or wrong decisions about your lifestyle choices and healthcare. The book offers insights into how you can make wiser decisions based on science to improve your health.

Gold Medal Winner, 2023 Nautilus Book Awards and
Independent Press (Ippy) Awards

New Insights Press

ISBN: 978-1-7359344-7-1 (Paperback)
ASIN: B09QV7GLQ5 (eBook)

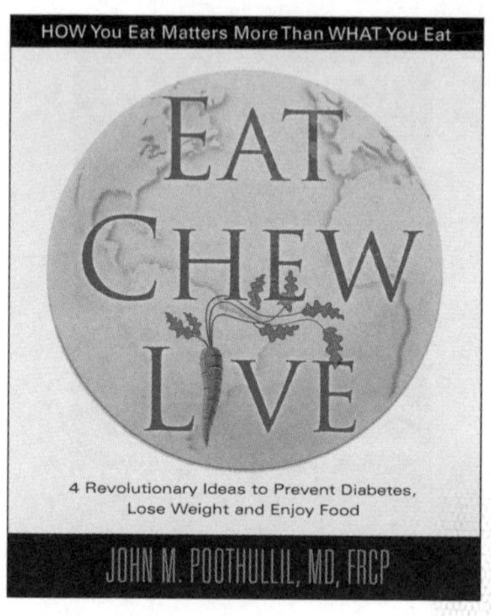

Eat Chew Live: 4 Revolutionary Ideas to Prevent Diabetes, Lose Weight and Enjoy Food

This book goes into extensive detail about the lack of logic with the insulin resistance theory as the cause of high blood sugar and Type 2 diabetes, and what everyone can do to change their thinking and eating habits.

Winner, 2016 Beverly Hills Books Awards

Over and Above Press

ISBN: 978-0-9907924-1-3 (Paperback)
ASIN: B0108UXZXA (eBook)